PREVENTIVE HEALTH SERVICES
FOR ADOLESCENTS

PREVENTIVE HEALTH SERVICES
FOR ADOLESCENTS

By

JOHN S. WODARSKI, Ph.D.

Associate Vice-President for Research
and Graduate Studies
The University of Akron
Akron, Ohio

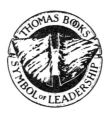

CHARLES C THOMAS • PUBLISHER
Springfield • Illinois • U.S.A.

Published and Distributed Throughout the World by

CHARLES C THOMAS • PUBLISHER
2600 South First Street
Springfield, Illinois 62794-9265

© *1989 by* CHARLES C THOMAS • PUBLISHER
ISBN 0-398-05542-4
Library of Congress Catalog Card Number: 88-24934

With THOMAS BOOKS *careful attention is given to all details of manufacturing
and design. It is the Publisher's desire to present books that are satisfactory as to their
physical qualities and artistic possibilities and appropriate for their particular use.*
THOMAS BOOKS *will be true to those laws of quality that assure a good name
and good will.*

Printed in the United States of America
Q-R-3

Library of Congress Cataloging in Publication Data

Wodarski, John S.
    Preventive health services for adolescents/by John S.
Wodarski.
        p.   cm.
    Includes bibliographies and index.
    ISBN 0-398-05542-4
    1. Preventive health services for teenagers. 2. Adolescent
psychology. I. Title.
    [DNLM: 1. Preventive Health Services--United States.
2. Psychology, Social--in adolescence. WS 462-W838p]
RJ101.W63 1989
362.2'0425'08805--dc19
DNLM/DLC
for Library of Congress   88-24934
                                                                CIP

CONTRIBUTORS

Pamela Harris, M.S.W.
Assessment Team Social Worker
Northeast Georgia Health District
Community Care Program
Athens, Georgia

Pamela Harris, at the time of her contribution to this text, was a research assistant at the University of Georgia School of Social Work Research Center while attending the graduate program in social work. Ms. Harris is now practicing social work with the Northeast Georgia Health District's Community Care Program in Athens.

Mitzi Hedrick, B.A.
Research Assistant
The University of Georgia
School of Social Work Research Center
Tucker Hall
Athens, Georgia

Mitzi Hedrick received her bachelor's degree in psychology at the University of Georgia and is currently enrolled in the master's program at the School of Social Work.

Lettie L. Lockhart, Ph.D.
Assistant Professor
The University of Georgia
School of Social Work
Tucker Hall
Athens, Georgia

Doctor Lettie Lockhart is an Assistant Professor at the University of Georgia School of Social Work and has collaborated with Doctor Wodarski on several grants and publications. She has written articles on teenage pregnancy, family violence, and children with AIDS, and currently serves on several local infant mortality and teenage pregnancy task forces. She was a 1987-1988 Lilly Teaching Fellow.

PREFACE

THE PREVENTION APPROACH to service has implications for the traditional role of the social worker and to the timing of the intervention. The major emphasis in prevention is on the teachig components of the intervention process. Social workers attempt to help clients learn how to exert control over their own behaviors and over the environments in which they live. Practitioners do not assume a passive role; instead, they use their professional knowledge, expertise and understanding of human behavior theory and personality development in the construction and implementation of intervention strategies. Since their training equips them to evaluate scientifically any treatment procedure they have instituted, there is continual assessment of the process.

Timing is a critical issue to be considered, as the helping professions traditionally have dealt with individuals only *after* the exhibition of problematic behaviors rather than *before* their occurrence. It is reasonable to question whether it is possible to alter clients' behaviors after 20, 40, or 60 years of learning. Our task, therefore, is to facilitate the preventive and educative roles that can be assumed by social workers. We should develop criteria for early intervention in terms of the age of the client, service context, and agent of change (Wodarski, 1987).

Prevention is especially appropriate to dealing with the problems of adolescents in America where the rates of teenage pregnancy, substance abuse, depression and subsequent suicide, violent behavior, and unemployment are higher than in any industrialized democracy (Estes, 1984; Murray, 1984). Problem behaviors of the young and their undesirable consequences are extensive and well documented. Teenagers' experimentation with drugs and alcohol can lead to overindulgence and abuse. Serious short- and long-term effects include risk taking and daredevil behavior that results in accidents, a leading cause of death among adolecents. Moreover, substance abuse among youth may increase the incidence of irresponsible sexual activity that results in venereal disease, unwanted pregnancy, and premature parenthood. Prevention efforts geared toward the adolescent developmental period would reduce these serious social problems. Prevention provides a view of the adolescent that is optimistic. The approach is mass-oriented rather than individual-oriented, and it seeks to build health from the start rather than to repair.

In the application of the prevention model to adolescents, the Life Skills Training approach is proposed as the treatment of choice. This paradigm has rationale and elements in common with other prevention programs that are based on a public health orientation. These programs consist of three essential components: (1) health education, (2) skills training, and (3) practice applying skills. The Teams-Games-Tournaments (TGT) model, a small group teaching technique with a substantial empirical history, is elucidated as an effective strategy for preventive intervention with adolescents. TGT emphasizes peers as teachers.

Prototypes of the preventive approach include courses on parental effectiveness, sex education, marital enrichment, and so on. Such courses focus on helping parents develop better communication and consistent child management skills, two variables research has shown are necessary conditions for successful child rearing (Hoffman, 1977; Patterson & Forgatch, 1987), and helping prepare young adults for the requisites of marriage, with effective communication skills, problem-solving strategies, and conflict resolution procedures (Collins, 1971; Ely, Guerney, & Stover, 1973; Lederer & Jackson, 1968; Rappaport & Harrell, 1972; Satir, 1967; Wodarski & Thyer, in press).

Prevention provides an early developmental focus for intervention that may forestall the onset of problems that intensify through time and become harder to alter. Prevention during the adolescent developmental period would reduce serious physical and social problems and thereby lessen the economic and emotional consequences to youth and their families. It is a difficult task for the practitioner to incorporate this new mode of practice, but it is a goal worthy of our attention. This text is devoted to helping the practitioner to address the problems of teenage pregnancy, substance abuse, depression and suicide, violent behavior, and preparation for the world of work, through the use of preventive interventions based on sound empirical data.

J.S.W.

REFERENCES

Collins, J. D. (1971). *The effects of the conjugal relationship modification method on marital communication and adjustment.* Unpublished doctoral dissertation, The Pennsylvania State University.

Ely, A.L., Guerney, G. G., & Stover, L. (1973). Efficacy of the training phase of conjugal therapy. *Psychotherapy: Theory, Research and Practice, 10,* 201-207.

Estes, R. J. (1984). *The social progress of nations.* New York: Praeger.

Hoffman, M. L. (1977). Personality and social development. In M. Rosenzweig, & L. Porter (Eds.), *Annual review of psychology* (pp.295-321). Palo Alto, CA: Annual Review.

Lederer, W., & Jackson, D. (1968). *The mirages of marriage.* New York: Morton.

Murray, C. (1984). *Losing ground: American social policy 1950-1980.* New York: Basic Books.

Patterson, G., & Forgatch, M. (1987). *Parents and adolescents living together. Part 1: The basics.* Eugene, OR: Castalia Publishing.

Rappaport, A., & Harrell, J. (1972). A behavioral exchange model for marital counseling. *The Family Coordinator, 21,* 203-212.

Satir, V. (1967). *Conjoint family therapy.* Palo Alto, CA: Basic Books.

Wodarski, J. S. (1987). *Social work practice with children and adolescents.* Springfield, IL: Charles C Thomas.

Wodarski, J. S., & Thyer, B. A. (in press). Behavioral perspectives on the family: An overview. In B. A. Thyer (Ed.), *Behavioral family interventions* (an edited volume in the NCFR/Sage Monograph Series).

CONTENTS

PREVENTIVE HEALTH SERVICES
FOR ADOLESCENTS

Chapter 1

ADOLESCENT DEVELOPMENT: A PREVENTIVE PERSPECTIVE

THE PREVENTION APPROACH to intervention has implications for the traditional role of the social worker and to the timing of the intervention. The prevention approach places major emphasis on the teaching components of the intervention process (Wodarski & Bagarozzi, 1979). Social workers attempt to help clients learn how to exert control over their own behaviors and over the environments in which they live. Practitioners do not take a passive role in the intervention process. Instead, they use their professional knowledge, expertise and understanding of human behavior theory and personality development in the conceptualization and implementation of intervention strategies. Since their training equips them to evaluate scientifically any prevention procedure they have instituted, there is continual assessment of the prevention process.

Prevention is especially appropriate to dealing with the problems of the adolescent. It provides an early developmental focus for intervention which may forestall development of future problems. These problems usually intensify later and become harder to alter in terms of time and money. Prevention provides a view of the person that is optimistic. The approach is mass-oriented rather than individual-oriented, and it seeks to build health from the start rather than to repair.

Problem behaviors of the young and their undesirable consequences are extensive and well documented. Teenagers' experimentation with drugs and alcohol can lead to overindulgence and abuse. Serious short- and long-term effects include risk-taking and daredevil behavior that increases risks to mental and physical health, including accidents—a leading cause of death among adolescents. Likewise, they may increase

the incidence of irresponsible sexual activity which eventuates in venereal disease, unwanted pregnancy, and premature parenthood. Prevention during the adolescent developmental period would reduce these
serious physical and social problems.

Initially, the chapter defines prevention and previews the three approaches to prevention: primary, secondary, and tertiary. From a life
span developmental approach, skills that an adolescent must master,
such as social, cognitive and academic, should provide the focus for intervention. The life skills approach is proposed as the treatment of
choice. This approach has rationale and elements in common with other
prevention programs that are based on a public health orientation.
These consist of three essential components: health education, skills
training, and practice applying skills. The teams-games-tournaments
model consists of the same components except that in addition it uses
peers as parallel teachers. The chapter reviews data available to support
the life skills and teams-games-tournaments model.

Prevention Defined

Whereas a major preoccupation of adolescent mental health programs across the country appears to be crisis intervention and direct
therapy, a more serious approach to reducing recurring problems, and
to detecting signs of future problems, is coming into focus. Proposed
programs, aimed at prevention, may be the key to mental health in the
1980s (Wodarski, 1983). Prevention is defined as the act of discouraging
a problematic behavior or illness before it actually happens or before it
becomes a problem. As there is a gradual shift away from the band-aid,
after-the-fact approach to mental health, programs designed to prevent
more serious consequences of present and/or future mental health problems or to prevent the recurrence of mental dysfunctioning are beginning to emerge in rural as well as in urban areas. Since it is more
cost-effective to prevent or reduce social problems, these programs proposed during a period of tight funds are sure to continue gaining appeal.

Social problems are the by-product of undesirable or ineffective behaviors. These behaviors frequently are the result of the adolescent's
failure to complete appropriate life span developmental tasks, and to attempt to cope with life's problems or to obtain desirable results when
attempts are made (D'Zurilla & Goldfried, 1971; Hughes, 1988).
Predisposing factors include economic distress, peer rejection, academic
failure, inadequate socialization, lack of problem-solving skills, racism,

and rapid physical changes (Whittman, 1977). These factors should be taken into account and dealt with as part of the problem gestalt.

Approaches to Prevention

Preventive programs should focus on those adolescents who will require services in the future if no ameliorating activities occur. The ultimate objective of preventive programs should be to eliminate or reduce the known predisposing factors within the community and thus reduce the number of adolescents at risk (Gottesfield, 1972). Preventive programs must teach alternate ways of dealing with environmental conditions (alternatives to undesirable behavior). For example, programs might focus on the development of social skills, or on acquisition of cognitive and emotional skills for reducing stress in one's own life (Rae-Grant, Gladwin, & Bower, 1966; Schinke & Blythe, in press). Essentially, preventive health programs must achieve two objectives. Each program must develop knowledge of factors that predispose the adolescent, and it must organize the community support systems to use this specific knowledge in its programs aimed toward altering such factors. Prevention of social distress encompasses, therefore, an array of programs, services and information.

Primary prevention is concerned with methods of reducing the overall incidence of social problems. Two foci of primary prevention which reduce the probability of interpersonal problems include teaching individuals to cope with stress and reducing stress in the actual environment (Gottesfield, 1972). Good examples of primary prevention of physical need deficits could be testing newborns for PKU to prevent mental retardation and providing adolescent parents information regarding child rearing. Primary prevention of lack of appropriate cognitive competencies should focus on acquisition of studying skills.

Secondary prevention takes on a different approach to the issue of social problems. Secondary prevention necessitates the organization of a helping system for selected candidates within the community (Caplan, 1974). Medication prescriptions for adolescents known to be distressed is an example of secondary prevention from a physical perspective. Secondary sociocultural prevention is present in school systems in the form of psychological testing and counseling services, and in mental health centers in the form of educational classes or groups to prevent substance abuse, depression and suicide among high-risk adolescents (Wodarski & Harris, 1985).

Tertiary prevention deals with adolescents who have had previous social problems. The goal is to maintain the individual in the community and to prevent problems from recurring. The effort here is to reduce the recidivism rate for adolescents who have been institutionalized. Community organization and planning is essential for tertiary prevention programs (Gottesfield, 1972). Tertiary prevention programs try to ensure that those who have recovered will be aided, not hampered, by the community to which they return (Caplan, 1961). Continued medication and referrals for additional services are examples of physical tertiary prevention services. Aftercare counseling, follow-ups, and day-treatment programs are all types of psychosocial tertiary prevention.

LIFE SPAN

A recent significant development in human behavior theory has been the life span development perspective (Wodarski, 1985). Its view is different from other human behavior theories in that it emphasizes a longitudinal approach. Its theorists emphasize that development occurs throughout life and that changes in the course of aging reflect biological, social, psychological, physical, and historical events, as well as the individual's activities as his/her own agent of change. At present, this view is shared by a significant number of practitioners. It is important for the social worker to be familiar not only with the life span perspective but also with the implications of each developmental stage for the client, the change agent, and subsequent practitioner interventions. Intervention efforts have been shown to be effective at every level of development, from birth through young adulthood, at which time the individual is unmalleable and difficult to treat due to "unresolved childhood conflicts." The life span approach posits that behavior and personality remain flexible throughout life and major changes can occur at any time. It suggests that many individuals have potential and untapped reserves that are infrequently recognized by change agents operating from more traditional models (Streever & Wodarski, 1984).

Early Adolescence (Thirteen to Seventeen Years)

The adolescent is preoccupied with rapid physical and intellectual maturation, heightened emotional sensitivity, and acceptance by social groups. Abstract thinking is possible and the adolescent is capable of conceptualizing changes that may occur in the future. The adolescent can anticipate the consequences of behavior and is especially sensitive to consistent and inconsistent parental behavior. Membership in peer groups that are more structured and organized than they were in earlier stages are extremely important. Group membership is most frequently based on physical attractiveness. The adolescent also begins engaging in heterosexual relationships. Parents and significant adults influence the child's identity and self-esteem less than the all-important peers.

The psychosocial crisis at this stage is "group identity versus alienation." The adolescent receives pressure from the parents, peers, and school to identify with a group. A positive resolution of the crisis results in the individual allying with a group that is perceived as meeting social needs and providing a sense of belonging. A negative resolution results in the adolescent experiencing a sense of isolation and continually feeling uneasy in the presence of peers. The central process is peer pressure (Newman & Newman, 1979).

Prevention Implications for the Worker. The worker needs to be concerned with the adolescent, the family, and the school. Families frequently seek treatment due to conflicted relationships at home. The family during this stage is at the point where the adolescent continues to meet parental expectations but gradually begins to assume a position as an adult. In families where parents are unhappy and in conflict, teenagers engage in high levels of rebellious and delinquent behaviors. Data indicate that if conflicts are not resolved, subsequent adolescent problems may develop (Feindler & Ecton, 1986). Parents who share decision making tend to have children who identify strongly with them. Parents who combine authority with reason and frequent communication tend to have adolescents who are assertive, responsible, and independent. These factors should be considered by the practitioner when working with families.

The peer group serves as a transitional world for the adolescent. Data suggest that participation in extracurricular activities is the most important determination of the adolescent's status with peers (Feldman, Caplinger, & Wodarski, 1983). The self-concept of the adolescent is very susceptible to status fluctuations that occur with family transiency and high school transitions. The worker should encourage the adolescent undergoing such transitions to become involved in extracurricular activities because they can provide support.

One of the most crucial problems workers will encounter is one of alcohol and drug abuse among teenagers. The substances become a problem when they are used by the adolescent to avoid the hard work that is required during this stage to achieve academic competencies and lasting social and psychological growth. In this situation, the worker should mobilize family, school, and community resources to abort the drug and alcohol abuse, including the use of Alcoholics Anonymous and Narcotics Anonymous groups for teenagers. Due to the prevalence of the problem, all communities and schools should provide education about alcohol and drugs for teenagers.

Later Adolescence (Eighteen to Twenty-Two Years)

During this psychosocial stage, individuals are primarily engaged in achieving autonomy from parents, with new peer groups having a substantial impact on their identity. Sex-role identity again becomes a major factor. The individual is also exploring his/her mortality and begins to perceive society's expectations for him/her. Turiel (1974) described this as a transitional stage where old principles are challenged and new ones have not yet emerged. This is the last stage before the individual has to make critical choices in terms of values, goals, and identity.

The individual also will be considering career alternatives. Frequently, he/she may feel that a choice must be made without much experience. Females may be strongly influenced by marriage and career expectations, and both males and females may make choices that reflect continued identification with parents. As the individual attempts to achieve autonomy, he/she may leave home and stop communicating with the family of origin for a time (Newman & Newman, 1979).

The psychosocial crisis during this stage is "identity versus role diffusion." The individual questions his/her essential character. Anxiety during this stage may encourage identity foreclosure, in which the individual makes choices based on others' expectations rather than experience the anxiety that accompanies forming his/her own identity (Marcia, 1966). Erikson (1959) posited that some individuals form negative identities that are based on social input (e.g. that one is "delinquent") or based on close identification with a negative role model. Role diffusion results when the individual is unable to integrate various roles or make a commitment to a single view of the self (Newman & Newman, 1979).

The central process of development during this stage is role experimentation. The individual may become involved in summer jobs, various religious and political groups, cohabitation, new peer groups, and so forth. Schenkel and Marcia (1972) reported that males become concerned with occupation and politics, whereas females are more likely to experiment with sexuality and religion. However, these differences may disappear as male and female liberation movements create more flexibility in roles.

World of Work. While youths' efforts to become employed are fraught with pain and frustration, the long-term effects of chronic unemployment on the mental health of these young persons are predictable and devastating. "Considering the magnitude of the problem and its deep psychological implications, the topic of unemployment in general has not received from social science researchers the attention that is deserved" (Sherraden & Adamek, 1983, p.2). Despite this limitation, however, existing studies do reveal consistent evidence and a fairly clear picture of the mental health aspects of unemployment.

It is critical to note the importance Americans place on employment and financial security. The Gallup organization (1980) conducted a study of adults in 1977 and another in 1980 and reported that the two most important problems facing their families at that time were economic and financial security, and unemployment. Unemployment is not simply an economic problem. It is also a psychological and sociological injury. Coles (1976) discovered that work was the most significant measure of "grown-up" status among working-class people.

Work has special meaning to the psychosocial development of young people. It is an opportunity to begin a career, to establish one's own identity, to gain independence, to contribute to family finances, to acquire prestige, and to try out adult roles. There is substantial research, for example, that indicates that for the majority of individuals, work is the single most defining aspect of living in American society. Conversely, unemployment at this age lowers feelings of self-esteem, and long spells of joblessness may precipitate catastrophic psychological problems. In Briar's study (1976) of youths, the impact of unemployment made them feel like they were "going crazy" and "suffocating." Some felt "mad at the whole world," "useless," "fed up," "stranded," and "incompetent and a failure." In addition to being bored, frightened, insecure, depressed and confused, some of them claimed their joblessness caused them to have problems with alcohol, eating and sleeping.

Increases in family conflicts were also reported. There are also indications that drug addiction, teenage pregnancy and family violence are related to youth joblessness (Dayton, 1978).

Associated with high unemployment rates are increases in homicides; motor vehicle mortality; residence in a mental hospital; and arrest rates for assault, criminal homicide, auto theft, robbery, rape, prostitution and narcotics (Brenner, 1980).

Despite high unemployment, the desire for jobs among youths in general, and among disadvantaged and minority youths in particular, remains strong (Briar, 1976). However, the job prospects for some youth are so bleak that after exhaustive unsuccessful job searches, they permanently drop out of the conventional labor force. They become alienated and disenfranchised from traditional social institutions. If not treated early, unemployment can have an irreversible impact on employment aspirations, social attachment and mental health.

The problem of youth unemployment is not simply a sign of the *present* economic times. Social and economic indicators forecast that youth joblessness may be a chronic problem. For example, even if the upturn in the economy continues, youth are competing for jobs with previously employed unemployed and with women and immigrants who are new to the job market. Furthermore, the high birth rates in the black population will continue to result in an increasing pool of black young people seeking to move into the job market.

Implications for the Social Worker. The social worker should have some knowledge of career alternatives and of the technologies available to help adolescents secure and maintain employment in order to assist the adolescent during this stage (Azrin & Victoria, 1980). The adolescent should be encouraged to engage in various work experiences and to consider both job security and job satisfaction in his/her final choice. Clients may need assistance from institutions, such as vocational rehabilitation, if they have not achieved adequate skills through traditional educational methods. At times, family treatment may be indicated if the individual is experiencing difficulty in becoming autonomous.

Turner (1976) stressed that treatment for the older adolescent having behavioral difficulties should utilize a multisystem approach that includes various community services in the treatment plan. This approach allows the individual to develop the numerous skills and the support systems that are necessary to achieve positive identity.

Peer Influence

For teenagers, actions detrimental to health frequently occur in situations involving peers. The influence of peer groups on adolescent behavior is well known (Sherif & Sherif, 1964) and, for many teenagers, strong social pressure provokes participation in peer-sanctioned behaviors such as smoking, abuse of substances, and sexual intercourse. Although teenagers may understand health risks involved in these activities, this understanding is insufficient to counter the social significance of indulging. Recent research (McAlister, Perry, & Maccoby, 1979) conducted jointly at Stanford and Harvard Universities underscores this point: "Behaviors detrimental to health are embedded in a complex milieu of social forces that often overwhelms educated rationality. . . . Even if a young person develops a negative attitude toward unhealthy behaviors, she or he may not possess the skills to resist strong social pressures to conform with peers who do not share that attitude." (p. 650).

Specific cognitive and behavioral skills are needed to resist external pressures and to successfully negotiate interpersonal encounters where pressure occurs. Adolescents often lack these skills not because of individual pathology but for developmental reasons. Age brings increased opportunity to engage in previously unknown or prohibited activities. Lack of experience and prior learning opportunities hamper youths' ability to deal with new situations and new behavioral requirements. Sexual experimentation provides an example. A significant number of 15-to17-year-olds in a recent national survey reported becoming sexually involved because it seemed "expected" of them and they did not know how to refuse (Cvetkovich & Grote, 1976; Forste & Heaton, 1988). Lack of interpersonal skill is also implicated in teenagers' frequent non-use of contraception (Kovar, 1979; Zelnik & Kantner, 1977). Recent research links failure to use contraception with failure to acquire critical assertive and communication skills (Campbell & Barnlund, 1977; Mindick, Oskamp, & Berger, 1978). These findings suggest teenagers may know about and value birth control, but, embarrassed and lacking skill, they may be unable to obtain it or to negotiate its use with sexual partners.

Similar inability to resist external pressure and lack of skill in handling critical interpersonal situations has been associated with onset of cigarette smoking (Newman, 1970) and drug and alcohol misuse (Roy & Shields, 1979; Smart, Gray, & Bennett, 1978). In short, a growing body of work suggests that teachers can profitably focus prevention and health promotion efforts on teaching youth skills for coping with risk-related interpersonal situations.

Progress in preventing health-impairing behavior is painfully slow (McAlister et al., 1979). Confusion exists as to what constitutes adequate prevention education (Matus & Neuhring, 1979). Therefore, primary educational prevention programs are poorly supported through policy and funding (Broskowski & Baker, 1977). In addition, because preventive educational intervention is frequently poorly designed, with vague goals compounding difficulties, prevention program effects are hard to evaluate, further diminishing the likelihood of public and legislative support. A new conceptualization is required if prevention and health promotion services are to become effective components of service systems.

There is an accurate data base to provide rationale and empirical support for the development of prevention and health education programs for adolescents. This is based on the Skills Training Interventive Model and the use of Teams-Games-Tournaments (TGT), a teaching method with a successful empirical history.

Skills Training Interventive Model[1]

The skills training model described here has rationale and elements in common with other preventive approaches based on a public health orientation (Caplan, 1964) and are variously called "graded pre-exposure" (Epstein, 1967), "immunization" (Henderson, Montgomery, & Williams, 1972), "psychological inoculation" (McGuire, 1964), "behavioral prophylaxis" (Poser, 1970, 1979), and "stress inoculation" (Meichenbaum, 1975). Whatever the label, the interventive goal is skill building to strengthen adolescents' resistance to harmful influences in advance of their impact. Three components comprise this preventive model: health education, skills training, and practice applying information and skills in troublesome situations.

Health Education

That adolescents need accurate information to make informed choices is clear. Equally clear is the inadequacy of simply exposing teenagers to facts about unhealthy consequences of certain behavior. One fault with past health education programs is their assumption that exposure to training materials guarantees learning. Information-only programs have had few long-lasting effects (Haggerty, 1977; Marsiglio & Mott, 1986). Accurate perception, comprehension, and storage of new information is a complex process dependent on individual receptivity and on the nature of the information presented (Mahoney, 1974). Particularly among younger adolescents, perceptual errors—selectively ignoring, misreading, or mishearing certain facts or selectively forgetting information—can create discrepancies between facts presented and facts received and remembered. The model proposed here addresses this potential problem by asking teenagers to periodically summarize presented content in written and verbal quizzes. Correct responses are then reinforced and errors detected and clarified. Also, peers are used as teachers, thus enhancing their commitment to healthy behaviors.

A second critical issue overlooked in traditional health education programs is helping youths relate specific facts and observable risks to themselves and to their own lives. Called "relational thinking" (Mahoney, 1974), this is the process by which abstract information becomes part of an individual's everyday reality. This relational or personalization process is best accomplished by actively involving adolescents in gathering and assimilating information. Examples include special information-collecting assignments (interviewing community resources and conducting mini-surveys) and experimental exercises requiring verbalization of facts and choices in personal terms ("Each time I have sex and don't use birth control, I risk pregnancy"). Also helpful for information personalization are direct discussions of illusions and faulty thinking patterns used to conveniently ignore important health facts (i.e. "It can't happen to me;" "I can quit anytime I want to;" "I never have an orgasm, so I don't have to worry about getting pregnant;" and the like).

Skills Training

Even personalized information is of little value if adolescents lack the skills to use it. Translating health information into everyday decision making and behavior involves cognitive and behavioral skills. The model thus emphasizes skills for making effective short- and long-term decisions and assertive and communication skills needed to implement decisions.

Cognitive skills training is adapted from research on problem solving (D'Zurilla & Goldfried, 1971; Spivack, Platt, & Shure, 1976). Especially for adolescents, problem behavior is associated with peer norms and expectations. Realistic decisions about how to act must, therefore, consider responses of significant others. The ability to anticipate both interpersonal and health consequences of behavior, generate alternative action strategies, and arrive at the best choice are all crucial to health-promotive decision making. Again, training focused on sexual behavior provides an example. Following discussion of birth control advantages and disadvantages, adolescents anticipate possible difficulties using this information in social situations; for instance, not knowing when or how to initiate discussion of birth control with dating partners. The problem is examined in detail and major issues identified, such as selecting appropriate times and places for discussion, handling personal embarrassment, and dealing with partner reactions. Adolescents generate several possible plans specifying when, where, and how the discussion could occur. They predict the probable outcome of each plan and select the one most feasible.

Training also focuses on behavioral skills necessary to transform decisions into action. Based on established assertive and communication skills-training procedures (Lange & Jakubowski, 1976; Schinke, Gilchrist, Smith, & Wong, 1976; Schinke & Rose, 1976), training presents verbal and non-verbal aspects of good communication to help adolescents learn to initiate difficult interactions, to practice self-disclosure of positive and negative feelings, to refuse unreasonable demands, to request changes in another's behavior, to ask others for relevant information and feedback, and to negotiate mutually acceptable solutions.

Practice Applying Skills

In the final and most important phase of the model, adolescents practice applying skills in a variety of potentially risky interpersonal situations. Extended role-played interactions provide adolescents with opportunities to recall and make use of health information, decision-making techniques, and communication skills as in the following vignette. You are at a party with someone you've been dating for about six months. The party is at someone's house; their parents are gone for the weekend. There is a lot of beer and dope and couples are going into the upstairs bedrooms to make out. Your date says, "Hey, Lisa and Tom have gone upstairs. It's real nice up there—let's go—come on."

In role playing, teenagers practice responding to increasingly insistent demands receiving feedback, instructions, and praise to enhance performance. Practice applying skills also takes the form of "homework" assignments involving written contracts to perform certain tasks outside the training environment such as meeting with a family planning counselor and initiating discussion of birth control with a dating partner.

Another example of applying skills is contained in the drug-refusal training aspects of the comprehensive health curriculum. The basic aim of drug-refusal training is to help students develop more effective ways of dealing with social pressures to consume drugs. Specific situations are practiced where individuals apply pressure to persuade others to consume excessive amounts of drugs. Students practice reactions to statements like: "One drink won't hurt you;" "What kind of friend are you;" or "Just have a little one, I'll make sure you won't have any more."

Components of appropriate reactions are taught such as: (1) to look directly at the pusher when responding; (2) to speak in a firm, strong tone with appropriate facial expressions and body language; (3) to offer an alternative suggestion such as "I don't care for a beer but I'd love a Coke"; (4) to request that the pushers refrain from continued persuasion; and (5) to change the subject by introducing a different topic of conversation.

Although all phases of the interpersonal skills training model can be conducted with individuals, groups provide the most efficient and effective training context for this final practice phase. Group settings allow teenagers to try out skills with various partners, give feedback and encouragement to each other, and learn from a variety of models.

Teams-Games-Tournaments Model

The most important socialization agent in an adolescent's life is his/her peers, with schools providing a natural environment for peer influence. Virtually all attempts to educate teenagers about health topics have taken an educational lecture model approach aimed at general education of all teenagers. Nearly all instruction in educational techniques are aimed at the individual pupil, ignoring the potential usefulness of the peer group in motivating students to learn and to acquire new skills or behaviors. Evaluative data indicate, however, the effectiveness of such an approach is minimal. Over the past three decades, a substantial amount of research has been conducted on learning groups. This research has suggested that learning teams in classrooms have uniformly positive effects on students.

The TGT technique, developed through two decades of research at the Johns Hopkins University Center for Social Organization of

Schools, is an innovative, small group teaching technique. The method is grounded in current theory, applies to diverse problems, populations, and settings, and provides clear criteria for evaluating program effects. The technique alters the traditional classroom structure and gives each student an equal opportunity to achieve and to receive positive reinforcement from peers by capitalizing on team cooperation, the popularity of games, and the spirit of competitive tournaments. Group reward structures set up a learning situation wherein the performance of each group member furthers the overall group goals. This has been shown to increase individual members' support for group performance, to increase performance itself under a variety of similar circumstances, and to further increase the group's goals. There is significance in using the group reward structure with adolescents, in that it capitalizes on peer influence and reinforcement, which are considered to be two of the most potent variables in the acquisition, alteration, and maintenance of prosocial behavior in youth (Buckholdt & Wodarski, 1978). Moreover, it facilitates the learning of low academic achievers who have low attachment to prosocial norms and peers, a group that is at greater risk to develop health problems. Data indicate that TGT is a viable mode for educating adolescents about health-related concerns. It has been found to be successful in helping children and adolescents acquire and retain knowledge in such areas as reading, arithmetic and social studies, and in the health-related areas.

Peer relationships play a significant role in the adolescent's socialization and health behavior. Thus, the information is provided in a group context to help students practice necessary social skills to develop adequate health behavior. Moreover, it capitalizes on the power of peers to influence the acquisition and subsequent maintenance of behavior which data indicate is the most potent influencing factor in an adolescent's life. It capitalizes on peers as teachers, and this changes the normative peer structure to support healthy behavior and increases the attachment high-risk peers have to prosocial norms and peers (Buckholdt & Wodarski, 1978).

Components of TGT Model

The components of the education program are as follows:

1. **Education.** This aspect includes facts about enhancing interpersonal relationships, alcohol and drugs, coping with sexuality, managing stress, promoting health, including good nutrition, securing employment, and accepting social responsibility.

2. **Self-Management.** The comprehensive educational program provides instruction in self-management. This component is based on social learning theory concepts. For example, students learn how certain stimuli cue drinking behavior such as parties, peer statements, emotional upset, and loneliness. Through assertiveness training, students are taught how to refuse alcohol in a socially acceptable manner. Additionally, they learn how to reward themselves for not drinking and for developing skills that will, in the future, bring them reinforcement.

Specific Preventive Activities

Many types of preventive activities can be undertaken. For example, in planning programs for adolescents the following topics can be included: (1) nutrition education; (2) social skills training; (3) adequate health care, i.e. smoking, sexuality, consumption of drugs; (4) job securement and maintenance; (5) resolving parental conflict; (6) problem-solving techniques; and (7) increasing self-esteem to reduce adolescent suicide. Programs are available to facilitate implementation of all of the above. For excellent reviews, see Gilchrist (1981), Hollin and Trower (1988), Schinke and Blythe (in press), Schinke, Blythe and Gilchrist (1981), Schinke, Gilchrist and Blythe (1980), Wodarski et al. (1980), Wodarski (1987, 1988), and Wodarski and Harris (1985).

In a more specific example, adolescents identified as high risk in terms of coping with the daily problems of living are taught a problem-solving approach based on the work of D'Zurilla and Goldfried (1971), Goldfried and Goldfried (1975), Schinke and Gilchrist (1984), and Spivack and Shure (1974). The general components emphasized are:

1. How to generate information
2. How to generate possible solutions
3. How to evaluate possible courses of action
4. Ability to choose and implement strategies through the following procedures:
   a. General introduction to how the provision of certain consequences and stimuli can control problem-solving behavior
   b. Isolation and definition of a behavior to be changed
   c. Use of stimulus control techniques to influence rates of problem-solving behavior
   d. Use of appropriate consequences to either increase or decrease a behavior

5. Verification of the outcome of the chosen course of action

Adolescents having difficulty in securing employment and social interaction could benefit from the two programs outlined below.

Vocational Enrichment Program

The vocational program is based on the work of Azrin (1978), Azrin, Flores and Kaplan (1975), and Jones and Azrin (1973). The general components emphasized are:

1. Group discussions involving strong motivation for vocational enrichment. These discussions involve mutual assistance among job seekers, development of a supportive buddy system, family support, sharing of job leads, and widening the variety of positions considered.

2. Employment securing aids, such as searching want ads, role playing, interview situations, instructions in telephoning for appointments, procedures for motivating the job seeker, developing appropriate conversational competencies, ability to emphasize strong personal attributes in terms of dress and grooming, and securing transportation for job interviews.

Social Enrichment Program

This program is based on the work of Lange and Jakubowski (1976) and involves interpersonal skills training and development of assertive behavior for appropriate situations. Specific elements that are emphasized include:

1. How to introduce oneself
2. How to initiate conversations and continue them
3. Giving and receiving compliments
4. Enhancing appearance
5. Making and refusing requests
6. Spontaneous expression of feelings
7. Appropriate use of non-verbal distance, body language, face, hand and foot movement, and smiling

SUMMARY

A major challenge to the community mental health approach is the question of the timing of intervention. Prevention places great emphasis on the teaching components of the interventive process, with social workers attempting to help clients learn how to exert control over their own behaviors and the environments in which they live.

In recognition of the critical role of prevention in improving the mental health of all citizens, it has been suggested that a special staff be set up in each mental health center just for prevention programs (Rae-Grant et al., 1966). Such a setup would be costly, but the impact in the long run would be substantial. The initial cost no doubt would be great, but relative to the cost of remedial programs, prevention should prove a bargain.

It is also important to note that many crises facing adolescents are as much a function of the environment as of the adolescent. Responsible social workers must keep abreast of social conditions and lobby for appropriate programs at the community, state, and federal levels to supplement the services they are able to offer as individuals. In our rapidly changing culture, myriad challenges will continue to confront us not only as social workers but as individuals, and we must meet these challenges responsibly. The life span development approach enables practitioners to anticipate future consequences for adolescents if they fail to master requisite competencies at each stage of development and to plan subsequent appropriate interventions in terms of assessing the individual's physical, psychological, and social attributes that will interact with his/her environment to facilitate the accomplishment of requisite developmental tasks in order to be successful in American society.

This chapter reviewed the critical area of prevention for adolescent dysfunctioning. Two empirically documented models for helping adolescents, life skills and teams-games-tournaments, are proposed and exemplary programs have been elaborated.

Chapter Two reviews requisites for the establishment, implementation, and evaluation of social work prevention programs for adolescents. Chapter Three elaborates the various requisites for structuring prevention services for adolescents and the various curriculums that are available. Chapter Four elucidates the dilemma of teenage pregnancies and the implications for prevention. Chapter Five reviews the staggering area of adolescent substance abuse. Chapter Six elucidates adolescent depression and suicide and reviews means of influences and prevention. Chapter Seven reviews a preventive paradigm for violent children. In Chapter Eight, a comprehensive employment preparation program of adolescents with developmental disabilities is elaborated. Chapter Nine deals with family supports that are necessary for prevention to be effective. The final chapter deals with issues in adolescent prevention.

ENDNOTE

1. The Skills Training Model was developed by Steven Schinke and colleagues at the University of Washington School of Social Work. For an elaboration, see Schinke, S., & Gilchrist, L. D. (1984). *Life skills counseling with adolescents.* Baltimore, MD: University Park Press.

REFERENCES

Azrin, N.H. (1978, November). *A learning approach to job finding.* Paper presented at The Association for Advancement of Behavior Therapy, Chicago.

Azrin, N. H., Flores, T., & Kaplan, S. J. (1975). Job-finding club: A group-assisted program for obtaining employment. *Behavior Research and Therapy, 13,* 17-27.

Azrin, N. H., & Victoria, A. (1980). *Job club counselor's manual.* Baltimore: University Park Press.

Brenner, M. H. (1980). Estimating the social costs of youth employment problems. In *A review of youth employment problems, programs and policies: The youth employment problem* (Vol. 1). Washington, DC: U. S. Government Printing Office.

Briar, K. H. (1976). *The effect of long-term unemployment on workers and their families.* DSW dissertation, The University of California at Berkeley.

Broskowski, A., & Baker, F. (1977). Professional, organizational, and social barriers to primary prevention. *American Journal of Orthopsychiatry, 44,* 707-719.

Buckholdt, D. R., & Wodarski, J. S. (1978). The effects of different reinforcement systems on cooperative behaviors exhibited by children in classroom contexts. *Journal of Research and Development in Education, 12,* 50-68.

Campbell, B. K., & Barnlund, D. C. (1977). Communication patterns and problems of pregnancy. *American Journal of Orthopsychiatry, 47,* 134-139.

Caplan, G. (1961). *Prevention of mental disorders in children.* New York: Basic Books.

Caplan, G. (1964). *Principles of preventive psychiatry.* New York: Basic Books.

Caplan, G. (1974). *Support systems in community mental health: Lectures on concept development.* New York: Behavioral Publications.

Coles, R. (1976). Work and self-respect. *Daedalus, 105*(4), 29-38.

Cvetkovich, G., & Grote, B. (1976, May). *Psychosocial development and the social problem of teenage illegitimacy.* Paper presented at the Conference on Determinants of Adolescent Pregnancy and Childbearing, Elkridge, MD.

Dayton, C. W. (1978). The dimensions of youth unemployment. *Journal of Employment Counseling,* March, 3-27.

D'Zurilla, T. J., & Goldfried, M. R. (1971). Problem solving and behavior modification. *Journal of Abnormal Psychology, 78,* 101-126.

Epstein, S. (1967). Toward a unified theory of anxiety. In B. Mahar (Ed.), *Progress in experimental personality research* (Vol.4). New York: Academic Press.

Erikson, E. H. (1959). The problem of ego identity. *Psychological Issues, 1*(1), 101-164.

Feindler, E. L., & Ecton, R. B. (1986). *Adolescent anger control: Cognitive-behavioral techniques.* New York: Pergamon Press.

Feldman, R. A., Caplinger, T. E., & Wodarski, J. S. (1983). *The St. Louis conundrum: The effective treatment of antisocial youths.* Englewood Cliffs, NJ: Prentice-Hall.

Forste, R. T., & Heaton, T. B. (1988). Initiation of sexual activity among female adolescents. *Youth & Society, 19*(3), 250-268.

Gallup Organization. (1980). *American families, 1980: A summary of findings.* Princeton, NJ: Author.

Gilchrist, L. D. (1981). Social competence in adolescence. In S. Schinke (Ed.), *Behavioral methods in social welfare* (pp. 61-80). New York: Aldine Publishing Co.

Goldfried, M., & Goldfried, A. (1975). Cognitive change methods. In F. Kanfer & A. Goldstein (Eds.), *Helping people change.* New York: Pergamon Press.

Gottesfield, J. (1972). *The critical issues of community mental health.* New York: Behavioral Publications.

Haggerty, R. J. (1977). Changing lifestyle to improve health. *Preventive Medicine, 6,* 276-280.

Henderson, A. S., Montgomery, I. M., & Williams, C. L. (1972). Psychological immunization: A proposal for preventive psychiatry. *Lancet, 13,* 1111-1112.

Hollin, C. R., & Trower, P. (1988). Development and applications of social skills training: A review and critique. In M. Hersen, R. Eisler, & P. Miller (Eds.), *Progress in behavior modification* (Vol. 22, pp. 166-214). Newbury Park, CA: Sage.

Hughes, J. N. (1988). *Cognitive behavior therapy with children in schools.* New York: Pergamon Press.

Jones, R. J., & Azrin, N. H. (1973). An experimental application of a social reinforcement approach to the problem of job finding. *Journal of Applied Behavior Analysis, 6,* 345-353.

Kovar, M. G. (1979). Some indicators of health-related behavior among adolescents in the United States. *Public Health Reports, 94,* 109-118.

Lange, A. J., & Jakubowski, P. (1976). *Responsible assertive behavior.* Champaign, IL: Research Press.

Mahoney, M. J. (1974). *Cognition and behavior modification.* Cambridge, MA: Ballinger.

Marcia, J. E. (1966). Development and maturation of ego identity status. *Journal of Personality and Social Psychology, 3,* 551-558.

Marsiglio, W., & Mott, F. L. (1986). The impact of sex education on sexual activity, contraceptive use and premarital pregnancy among American teenagers. *Family Planning Perspectives, 18*(4), 151-162.

Matus, R., & Neuhring, E. M. (1979). Social workers in primary prevention: Action and ideology in mental health. *Community Mental Health Journal, 15,* 33-40.

McAlister, A. L., Perry, C., & Maccoby, N. (1979). Adolescent smoking: Onset and prevention. *Pediatrics, 63,* 650-658.

McGuire, W. J. (1964). Inducing resistance to persuasion: Some contemporary approaches. In L. Berkowitz (Ed.), *Advances in experimental social psychology* (Vol. 1). New York: Academic Press.

Meichenbaum, D. (1975). Self-instructional methods. In F. Kanfer & A. Goldstein (Eds.), *Helping people change.* New York: Pergamon Press.

Mindick, B., Oskamp, S., & Berger, D. E. (1978, August). *Prediction of adolescent mental health.* Paper presented at the meeting of the American Psychological Association, Toronto, Canada.

Newman, B. M. (1970). Peer pressure hypothesis for adolescent cigarette smoking. *School Health Review, l,* 15-18.

Newman, B. M., & Newman, P. R. (1979). *Development through life: A psychosocial approach.* Homewood, IL: Dorsey.

Poser, E. G. (1970). Toward a theory of "behavioral prophylaxis." *Journal of Behavior Therapy and Experimental Psychiatry, l,* 39-43.

Poser, E. G. (1979). Issues in behavioral prevention: Empirical findings. *Advances in Behavior Research and Therapy, 2,* 1-25.

Rae-Grant, Q. A. F., Gladwin, T., & Bower, E. M. (1966). Mental health, social competence, and war on poverty. *American Journal of Orthopsychiatry, 36,* 652-664.

Roy, T., & Shields, R. (1979). Alcohol education in school social work. *Social Work in Education, 1,* 43-53.

Schenkel, S., & Marcia, J. E. (1972). Attitudes toward premarital intercourse in determining ego-identity status in college women. *Journal of Personality, 3,* 472-482.

Schinke, S. P., & Blythe, B. J. (in press). Cognitive-behavioral prevention of childrens' smoking. *Child and Behavior Therapy.*

Schinke, S. P., Blythe, B. J., & Gilchrist, L. D. (1981). Cognitive-behavioral prevention of adolescent pregnancy. *Journal of Counseling Psychology, 28,* 451-454.

Schinke, S. P., & Gilchrist, L. D. (1984). *Life skills counseling with adolescents.* Baltimore: University Park Press.

Schinke, S. P., Gilchrist, L. D., & Blythe, B. J. (1980). Role of communication in the prevention of teenage pregnancy. *Health and Social Work, 5,* 54-59.

Schinke, S. P., Gilchrist, L. D., Smith, T. E., & Wong, S. E. (1976). Group interpersonal skills training in a natural setting: An experimental study. *Behavior Research and Therapy, 17,* 149-154.

Schinke, S. P., & Rose, S. D. (1976). Interpersonal skills training in groups. *Journal of Counseling Psychology, 23,* 442-448.

Sherif, M., & Sherif, C. W. (1964). *Reference groups: Exploration into conformity and deviation of adolescents.* New York: Harper & Row.

Sherraden, M. W., & Adamek, M. (1983). Unemployment and adolescent mental health. *Practice Applications, 1,* 1-15.

Smart, R. G., Gray, G., & Bennett, C. (1978). Predictors of drinking and signs of heavy drinking among high school students. *The International Journal of the Addictions, 13,* 1079-1094.

Spivack, G., Platt, J. J., & Shure, M. B. (1976). *The problem-solving approach to adjustment.* San Francisco: Jossey-Bass.

Spivack, G., & Shure, M. B. (1974). *Social adjustment of young children.* San Francisco: Jossey-Bass.

Streever, K. L., & Wodarski, J. S. (1984). Life span development approach: Implications for practice. *Social Casework, 65*(5), 267-278.

Turiel, E. (1974). Conflict and change in adolescent moral development. *Child Development, 45*(1), 14-29.

Turner, F. J. (Ed). (1976). *Differential diagnosis and treatment in social work.* New York: Free Press.

Whittman, M. (1977). Application of knowledge about prevention in social work education and practice. *Social Work and Health Care, 3,* 37-47.

Wodarski, J. S. (1983). *Rural community mental health practice.* Austin, TX: PRO-ED.

Wodarski, J. S. (1985). *Introduction to human behavior.* Austin, TX: PRO-ED.

Wodarski, J. S. (1987). Evaluating a social learning approach to teaching adolescents about alcohol and driving: A multiple variable evaluation. *Journal of Social Service Research, 10,* 121-144.

Wodarski, J. S. (1988). Teams-games-tournaments: Teaching adolescents about alcohol and driving. *Journal of Alcohol and Drug Education, 33*(3), 46-57.

Wodarski, J. S., & Bagarozzi, D. (1979). A review of the empirical status of traditional modes of interpersonal helping: Implications for social work practice. *Clinical Social Work Journal, 7*(4), 231-255.

Wodarski, J. S., & Harris, P. (1985). Adolescent suicide: A review of influences and the means for prevention. *Practice Applications, 2*(4). (A publication of the Washington University Center for Adolescent Mental Health, St. Louis, MO).

Wodarski, L. A., Adelson, C., Tidball, M., & Wodarski, J. S. (1980). Teaching nutrition by teams-games-tournaments. *Journal of Nutrition Education, 12*(2), 61-65.

Zelnik, M., & Kantner, J. F. (1977). Sexual and contraceptive experience of young unmarried women in the United States, 1976 and 1971. *Family Planning Perspectives, 9,* 55-71.

Chapter 2

REQUISITES FOR THE ESTABLISHMENT, IMPLEMENTATION AND EVALUATION OF SOCIAL WORK PREVENTION PROGRAMS FOR ADOLESCENTS

MANY SOCIAL WORK researchers, theorists, and practitioners have called for the establishment of social work. services on a more rational basis and for the empirical evaluation of services in order to assess whether needs of children and adolescents are being adequately met (Brown, 1968; Fischer, 1973a, 1973b; Geismar, LaGay, Wolock, Gerhart, & Fink, 1972; Handler, 1975; Henderson & Shore, 1974; Lipton, Martinson, & Wilks, 1975; Meyer, Borgatta, & Jones, 1965; Mullen & Dumpson, 1972; Lundman, 1976; Lundman, McFarlane, & Scarpitti, 1976; Reid & Shyne, 1969; Sarri & Selo, 1974; Schinke & Gilchrist, 1984; Schwartz, 1966, 1971; Voit, 1975; Wodarski & Pedi, 1977). A review of the literature, however, reveals little consideration of steps involved in the planning and implementation of prevention programs and their subsequent evaluation. It is more unfortunate that steps involved in the evaluation of programs tend to be elaborated without regard to the procedures involved in establishing and implementing them. Indeed, implementation and evaluation are interrelated. Adequate evaluation of services is not practicable without meeting key requisites for the establishment and implementation phases of social work prevention programs. Thus, the central aim of this chapter is to discuss basic requisites for planning, implementing and evaluating social work prevention programs for adolescents.

Recent research investigations provide data to suggest that many interventions and treatment contexts are inappropriate for the provision of services (Feldman, Caplinger, & Wodarski, 1983). For example, in most treatment programs for adolescents there occur crucial dysfunctions as a result of homogeneously grouping antisocial adolescents together for the purposes of treatment. Moreover, most programs provide interventions in social contexts other than those where the problematic behaviors first, or most frequently, occur. Thus, even if prosocial behaviors are learned during the course of treatment, the capacity to generalize such learned behaviors to the open environment is unduly limited. Likewise, in such treatment contexts the labeled client typically receives services along with others who are similarly defined, thereby increasing the likelihood that the adolescent will acquire a more negative and stigmatizing label. As certain researchers suggest, this may lead toward establishment of a deviant self-concept and/or deviant identity. Also, in such settings the client is less likely to be provided the opportunity to view adequate role models. Interaction with normal peers is severely constrained, and role models provided in segregated treatment milieus may be more deviant than those provided in other treatment settings, thus diminishing the likelihood of positive reinforcement from peers for prosocial behaviors (Feldman et al., 1983). Moreover, the timing of interventions are too late to be effective in terms of costs.

This presentation focuses initially on a series of major prevention considerations. What is the appropriate context for behavioral change? Who should act as the change agent? What characteristics should he/she possess? What are the rationales for service provided? How long should interventions continue? How does one prepare for the termination of interventions? How does one ensure that behaviors acquired in interventions are maintained, and so forth? The discussion also will focus on the organizational factors of contexts of interventions which are pertinent to the creation of services, structural components and the training of staff. Finally, the chapter reviews the characteristics of efficacious prevention programs for adolescents and a number of requisites for the adequate evaluation of these programs. Specific items discussed are: securing an adequate baseline of behaviors; specifying the behaviors to be changed; specifying workers' behaviors in terms of relationship formation and intervention; measures of worker and client behavior; specification of criteria for evaluation of prevention efficacy; monitoring of prevention implementation; and reliability of measures, designs and statistics applicable to evaluation, follow-up, implementation of findings, and so forth. Throughout the chapter relevant future research issues are reviewed.

Implementation of Change Strategy: By Whom, and How Long? Context of Behavioral Change

Unfortunately, if an adolescent exhibits a problematic behavior in a social context such as a school, the behavioral change strategies all too frequently are provided in another social context, such as a child guidance clinic, family service agency, community mental health center, and so forth. Such procedures create many structural barriers to effective intervention (Kazdin, 1977; Stokes & Baer, 1977). Therapeutic change should be provided in the same contexts where the problematic behaviors are exhibited. If therapeutic strategies are implemented in other contexts, the probabilities are reduced that newly learned behaviors can be sufficiently generalized and maintained. Considerable study is needed to delineate those variables that facilitate the generalization and maintenance of behavior change. These may include substituting "naturally occurring" reinforcers, training relatives, peers or other significant individuals in the client's networks, gradually removing or fading the contingencies, varying the conditions of training, using different schedules of reinforcement, using delayed reinforcement and self-control procedures, and so forth (Kazdin, 1975). Such procedures will be employed in future sophisticated and effective social service delivery systems.

By Whom Should Change Be Delivered?

We have little evidence to suggest what personal characteristics of change agents facilitate the delivery of services to adolescents. One could propose certain general hypotheses, e.g. workers should be reinforcing individuals with whom adolescents can identify; they should possess empathy, unconditional positive regard, interpersonal warmth, verbal congruence, confidence, acceptance, trust, verbal ability, physical attractiveness; and so forth (Carkhuff, 1969, 1971; Carkhuff & Berenson, 1967; Corrigan, Dell, Lewis, & Schmidt, 1980; Fischer, 1975; Suinn, 1974; Truax & Carkhuff, 1967; Wells & Miller, 1973; Vitalo, 1975; Wodarski, 1985). Likewise, Rosenthal (1966) and Rosenthal and Rosnow (1969) have suggested the workers' expectations of positive change in clients is also necessary. Additional research suggests that a behavioral change agent should have considerable verbal ability, should be motivated to help others change, should possess a wide variety of social skills, and should have adequate social adjustment (Berkowitz & Graziano, 1972; Garfield, 1977; Gruver, 1971). Even though other social science disciplines are beginning to gather preliminary data concerning the attributes and skills of helping agents, there is virtually no literature in the field of social work to indicate what type of characteristics a worker should possess in order to help adolescents. Presently, such decisions are made quite arbitrarily. The notion that professional training enables all workers to be equally effective in producing behavioral change is yet to be substantiated. Much more research is needed to delineate the characteristics of effective change agents. Thereafter, hopefully, schools of social work will be able to develop more appropriate selection measures and to create more effective educational technologies to facilitate the acquisition of requisite skills and attributes.

If a worker chooses to employ an adolescent's parents, teachers, peers, or others as change agents, he/she will have to assess at the very least how motivated these individuals are to help alleviate the dysfunctional behavior, how consistently they will apply change techniques, what means are available to monitor the implementation of interventions to ensure that it is appropriately applied, and if the chosen change agent possesses characteristics such as similar social attributes, similar sex, and so forth that could facilitate the client's identification with the worker (Bandura, 1969, 1977; Tharp & Wetzel, 1969).

Assessment

The crucial question of who should be exposed to intervention centers on adequate assessment. Assessment must be of a reliable and valid nature to ensure a minimal number of false positives. Thus, multiple criteria of measurement should be utilized in terms of self-inventories, interviews, and behavioral observation. Moreover, the data should be secured from as many different data bases as possible.

Rationale for Prevention Services Provided

The rationale for offering a program should be based primarily on empirical grounds. The decision-making process should reflect that the change agents have considered what type of agency should house the service, that they have made an assessment of the organizational characteristics of the intervention context, and that the interests of agency personnel have been considered in planning the service. A number of additional questions also should be posited. How can the program be implemented with minimal disruption? What new communication structures need to be added? What types of measurements can be used in evaluating the service? What accountability mechanisms need to be set up? What procedures can be utilized for monitoring execution of the program (Wodarski & Feldman, 1974)?

Duration

No empirical guidelines exist regarding how long a service should be provided, that is, when client behavior has improved sufficiently, in terms of quality and quantity, to indicate that services are no longer necessary. Such criteria should be established before the service is to be provided and these should indicate how the program will be evaluated. The criteria should enable workers to determine whether or not a service is meeting the needs of the client. Moreover, they should help reveal the particular factors involved in deciding whether or not a service should be terminated. The more concrete the criteria, the less this process will be based on subjective factors.

ORGANIZATIONAL FACTORS PERTINENT TO THE CREATION OF PREVENTION SERVICES FOR ADOLESCENTS

Structural Components

Few agencies have considered the key organizational requisites for the evaluation of prevention services. In fact, most agencies are physically structured in a suboptimum manner for the delivery or evaluation of prevention. For example, few agencies provide observational areas with *one-way mirrors* where therapists can observe each other and isolate effective techniques for working with an adolescent or his/her family unit. Viewing areas enable the unobtrusive gathering of samples of an adolescent's behavior and facilitate the recording of interaction between parents and the adolescent. They can facilitate training programs where parents learn to change interactional patterns with their adolescent, and they can provide a means by which parents can view and model behaviors which the therapists exhibit in working with the adolescent and sharpen appropriate social skills. These measures also may enable workers to secure necessary data for the systematic evaluation of preventive services. The provision of such feedback to workers enables them to sharpen their practice skills, adds to practice knowledge, and provides another vehicle for teaching practice skills.

Another technological advance that will be of considerable help in evaluating the services provided to children is the use of *videotapes*. Videotapes can document many verbal and non-verbal interactions. They can provide a more effective and reliable medium through which preventive services can be evaluated. Likewise, with proper analysis they can help to sharpen practice skills and lead to a better understanding of how verbal and non-verbal behaviors exhibited by clients and workers influence their mutual interactions and facilitates the use of appropriate models to facilitate acquisition of relevant behaviors (Wodarski, 1975).

Training of Change Agents

Literature is just beginning to accumulate on the procedures that should be utilized in the training of change agents. One relevant training program has been developed on a pilot basis by the author (Wodarski, 1974). It has evolved as part of an evaluative research project regarding the assessment of a community-based treatment program for antisocial children. The training program consisted of initially presenting to students the basic rationale for using a social learning model in training change agents, that is, it permits objectives to be clearly operationalized and measured. During the training process the students gained an in-depth knowledge of social learning principles through extensive reading. Second, three essential elements were reviewed which form the foundation of the training process: the operationalization of preventive interventions (behaviors to be exhibited by the change agent), and the acquisition of data to determine if the isolated events chosen to alter the client's behaviors (antecedents and consequences) have influenced the rate of the adolescent's behavior. Next, students were exposed to observational scales used to measure client and change agents' behaviors and to experimental designs that they could implement to evaluate their practice behavior. The incorporation of this knowledge in their subsequent training was used to demonstrate such techniques as reinforcement, modeling of appropriate behaviors, punishment, and so forth. Videotapes of professionals and students simulating small group interaction where they practiced the application of interventive techniques were used in order to help the change agents acquire requisite practice behaviors. It also was emphasized how periodic feedback from practitioners and students can enhance learning and practice skills. Before work with a client was initiated, the students were required to review a tape of clients interacting in a group, to make an assessment, to design a corresponding prevention plan, and to specify how the success of the prevention would be determined (Wodarski, 1985).

EVALUATION AND CHARACTERISTICS OF AN EFFICACIOUS PREVENTION PROGRAM FOR ADOLESCENTS

Adequate Specification of Behaviors and Baselines

An adequate prevention program must take into account the need for reliable specification of target behaviors; that is, those behaviors which are to be changed. For example, a prevention program to alleviate antisocial behavior might employ behavioral rating scales where the deviant behaviors are concretely specified. These could include such observable behaviors as hitting others, damaging physical property, running away, climbing and jumping out of windows, making loud noises and aggressive or threatening verbal statements, throwing objects, such as paper, candy, erasers, chairs, and so forth.

A prerequisite for the adequate evaluation of any preventive service is to secure a baseline prior to implementation of prevention. This enables the investigator to asess how his/her preventive interventions compare with **no** preventive interventions. The best type of baseline measure is secured by behavioral observers, who generally have learned to establish reliability on behavioral categories through an extensive training procedure. If observations of behaviors cannot be secured by trained observers, there are other less desirable data sources, such as baselines taken by the client him/herself or by significant others in his/her environment. Even though less reliable, these baselines many times are necessary due to various organizational or other environmental constraints. Some of these constraints may involve lack of money for trained observers or the investigation of a behavior that occurs at a time when it is not readily observable by others. When the researcher uses baseline data not secured by a trained observer, the data should be obtained from two or more independent sources in order to check on consistency.

The following are various practical considerations that should be addressed before a researcher decides on the exact procedures for securing a baseline. The first consideration involves where the baseline should be taken. A context should be chosen in which the individual's behavior occurs at a high frequency. If the behavior occurs in more than one context, baselines may be secured for the various contexts. This enables the assessment of a broader range of contexts where the behavior occurs, contributes to the determination of whether or not behavioral changes in one context are analogous to those in another, and provides a more accurate measure of behavior. Additional considerations pertain to where the behavior occurs. If the behavior is readily accessible to observation, there will be no problem. If it is inaccessible, such as a behavior that occurs late at night or in contexts where observation is not possible, the investigator will have to use reports by the client, or others who are present when the behavior occurs, to secure the data. As previously mentioned, it is preferable to have a trained observer secure data. In any case, an individual who is consistent and reliable should be chosen, and data should be collaborated in instances where this is possible. Finally, whether the person who secures data is a trained observer or someone else, a necessary requisite for evaluation of the service is the execution of periodic reliability checks to ensure that the data being provided are consistent (Nelson, Lipinski, & Black, 1975).

Characteristics of Control Groups

Much of the controversy in human services centers on whether or not services offered clients significantly affect their lives. Control groups are necessary to isolate whether interventions were effective and to provide data to resolve this controversy.

Ideally, two control groups should be used in research conducted to evaluate services: a waiting list control and an active control group. An active control group provides a baseline rate of improvement or deterioration over time to which the experimental intervention can be compared and evaluated. To provide an accurate comparison, this control group should contain all the essential features of the intervention group except for the variables under investigation. For example, if we are evaluating social skills training, the control group should be similar in terms of worker expectations for change, testing procedures, and context and length of sessions. An active control group provides a refined analysis of the components of effective intervention. However, such a fine analysis may be too costly in terms of time, energy, and administrative execution. A waiting list control group isolates the number of clients who improve through the passage of time without receiving documented professional help. Although the employment of an active control group is preferable, a waiting list control group is the minimal prerequisite for the adequate evaluation of prevention effects. Both groups should be offered services immediately after the collection of requisite data.

Conceptualization and Operationalization of Intervention

Appropriate conceptualization and operationalization of interventions are imperative for the development of effective programs. A worker must be able to specify what behaviors he/she will implement in order to apply a given prevention strategy. This represents a difficult requirement for many, if not most, theoretical frameworks. Usually, prevention services are described on a global level and are assigned a broad label such as parent training, social skills training, stress inoculation, and so forth. However, such labels are valuable only so long as they specify the operations involved in implementing the services. For instance, the global label of social skills can be separated into the following distinct behavioral acts: problem solving, anger control, relaxation, and appropriate personal behaviors such as praise, position attention, holding, criticism, threats, appropriate eye contact, and so forth (Wodarski,1987). Moreover, essential attributes of the change agent that facilitate the implementation of interventions should be delineated.

Measures of Worker and Client Behavior

Various measures, such as checklists filled out by children and/or significant others (e.g. group leaders, parents, referral agencies, grandparents, and so forth) and behavioral time sampling schedules, can be utilized to assess change in adolescents. Likewise, behavioral rating scales can be used to assess the behaviors exhibited by a change agent. There are excellent texts available which describe the various measures that can be used.[1] They specify particular items measured and the appropriate clientele, types of data provided, reliability, and procedures involved in administration. The type of measurement process selected generally will depend upon the behaviors chosen for alteration, the availability of technical equipment, the cost of securing various types of data, the context of measurement, and the frequency, duration and intensity of the target behavior (Bijou, Peterson, Harris, Allen, & Johnston, 1969).[2]

The literature over the last decade has called for the utilization of multicriterion measurement processes for the evaluation of prevention services. However, the few investigators who have utilized multicriterion measurement indicate that many changes secured on certain inventories do not correspond necessarily with results of other measurement processes utilized. For example, in studies by Wodarski et al. (1975, 1976a, 1976b, 1988), it was found that little correlation exists between self-inventory and behavioral rating scales. In many instances, a change can occur on one of the measurements and not on another. The strongest data are derived from behavioral observation scales, simply because observers are trained for long periods of time to secure reliable and accurate data. If an appropriate behavioral observation scale is not available, then the investigator can develop his/her own scale by observing adolescents systematically and then accurately defining the relevant behaviors so that two people can consistently agree that they have occurred.

Both self-inventories and behavioral scales have certain drawbacks. Self-inventories have low reliability but they cost less; also, they may measure behavioral tendencies that behavioral scales do not measure. Behavioral scales provide highly reliable data but are more costly and, depending on the breadth of observation, they may provide data that are limited to a specific social context. The decision to utilize a particular measurement process rests on the aims of the research project.

Specification of Criteria for Evaluation of Prevention Efficacy

Any prevention program should specify the criteria by which the service will be evaluated. This should be done **before** the intervention is implemented. For example, evaluation may occur by means of behavioral observations provided by trained observers and/or through the use of checklists filled out by adolescents and significant others. In view of the multidimensional nature of human behavior, it seems necessary for professionals to evaluate more than a single criterion in order to develop a comprehensive and rational basis for the provision of services. Moreover, highly sophisticated intervention programs will endeavor to quantify the extent of behavioral change targeted and actually achieved and the social relevance of changes that have occurred; that is, do they really matter in terms of the client's ability to function in his/her environment (Kazdin, 1977)?

Intervention Monitoring

Having met all prior prerequisites, it then becomes necessary to monitor the implementation of interventions. Such monitoring should take place throughout services so that necessary adjustments can be made over time if the quality of the interventions vary. If behavioral change is obtained and if the investigator can provide data to indicate that interventions were differentially implemented, the change agents can claim with confidence that their services had been responsible for the observed modifications in behavior. However, if such data cannot be provided when client change has occurred, many rival hypotheses can be postulated to account for the results (Wodarski & Pedi, 1977).

Reliable Measures

Reliability must be secured for all measures utilized in evaluating a program. Without this basic scientific requisite, evaluative efforts may be ill-spent and there can be no assurance of consistency in the data secured. The reliability requirement often is disregarded in evaluative research, thus allowing for the postulation of rival hypotheses to account for the findings (Wodarski & Buckholdt, 1975).

Designs

Frequently, it has been assumed that the only way that intervention services can be evaluated is through the employment of classical experimental designs, e.g. those where participants are assigned randomly to one or more experimental or control groups. However, such designs may have many deficits and may not be the most appropriate for the evaluation of services. They may be expensive in terms of money, energy required to implement them and administration (Wodarski & Buckholdt, 1975). Moreover, the criterion of random assignment of subjects is usually hard to meet in the evaluation of services provided to adolescents. New designs, however, are emerging from social learning theory literature. These can be easily implemented in social work; they are economical in terms of money, energy required to implement them, and administrative execution. Above all, they provide data which will enable a worker to determine if his/her interventions have had an effect on client behaviors.

It is interesting to note that the emphasis in the evaluation of services in social work has been on the use of traditional experimental designs which involve grouping clients into experimental and control groups.

This research philosophy is diametrically opposed to a basic practice assumption, namely, that every individual is unique and needs to be considered in his/her own gestalt. The *single case* study, which has been championed in recent social learning research, may alleviate many of the measurement problems discussed. In this approach the client serves as his/her own control, and a client's change is evaluated against data provided by him/herself during a baseline period which precedes the application of intervention. This type of methodology also alleviates the moral and legal aspects of placing a client in a no-treatment control group. It is too early to predict the effects of various legal decisions on the use of traditional control groups in evaluative research. The use of these may be challenged in the future on two legal bases: (1) denial of the right to intervention, and (2) denial of equal protection (Wodarski, 1980).

The data provided in Figure 2-1 provide an example of a time-series design used to evaluate group work service provided to 10 five- and six-year-old antisocial children. In this figure percentage frequencies of prosocial, non-social and antisocial behavior are graphed for a group of children who met for two-hour sessions over a period of 14 weeks at a community center. This classical design in social learning theory consists of four basic phases and is commonly referred to as the ABAB design. In the first phase the children are exposed to a *baseline period*. During this period the group worker does not rationally plan interventions that are likely to influence the prosocial, non-social, or antisocial behavior within the group. This is analogous to a traditional diagnostic technique postulated by Sallie Churchill (1965), where the group worker refrains from interventions so that he/she can more accurately determine the treatment needs of the group. After the children's observed incidences of antisocial behavior have stabilized, treatment is begun (Phase II). Behaviors are considered stabilized if the average variance of the last session is within ten percentage points of the mean of the previous two or three sessions. Members' behaviors are monitored until they once again stabilize, whereupon a baseline condition is reintroduced (Phase III, or the reversal period). The procedure enables the therapist and others who evaluate the treatment program to determine whether the intervention itself was responsible for the various changes in behavior. Immediately after it becomes evident that the intervention has been effective in reducing antisocial behavior, the procedures are applied once again.

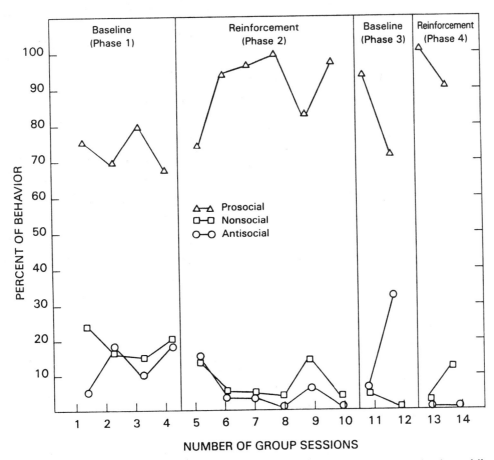

Figure 2-1. Average percentage of prosocial, non-social, and antisocial behavior exhibited by 10 children, according to number of group sessions.

In some situations the ABAB design may not be feasible due to the types of behaviors being modified and/or for various ethical reasons. The primary reason for utilizing an alternate design is that in the ABAB design the modified behavior usually will not reverse itself and, in many instances, reversals would be too damaging to the client or significant others. For example, when fighting is brought under control in a home it would not be feasible to do a reversal of this behavior since, in the past, undue physical harm may have been inflicted on others. A design that may be utilized in lieu of the ABAB design is the multiple baseline design, where a series of behaviors for modification are operationalized. Predictions are made regarding how the various techniques will affect different behaviors. Each behavior is then modified according to a time schedule. Usually, one or two behaviors are modified at a time. For example, the worker might want to decrease such behaviors as yelling, fighting, throwing objects, or straying from the group, and to increase prosocial behaviors, such as task participation, appropriate verbal comments, and so forth. The worker in this instance might choose first to ignore the yelling and to use positive reinforcement to increase appropriate verbal comments. Once the yelling decreases and the appropriate verbal comments increase, he/she would sequentially modify the second, third, and fourth behaviors. In Table 2-1 an outline is provided regarding how such a process operates. The technique being employed becomes more efficacious each time the behaviors change in the direction predicted for each child. This replication of results increases the practitioner's confidence in his techniques and is necessary in evaluative research, since the conclusions gained from any one study or interventive attempt are always considered tentative.

Table 2-1

MULTIPLE BASELINE DESIGN ACCORDING TO PHASES

Communication Problem	Day					
	1	4	8	14	19	109
Name	Baseline	Intervention			Follow-up I	Follow-up II
Function	Baseline	Baseline	Intervention		Follow-up I	Follow-up II
Command	Baseline	Baseline	Baseline	Intervention	Follow-up I	Follow-up II

Another design which can be used is the AB design. In actuality, it is the first half of the ABAB design. It involves securing a baseline and introducing treatment after the behavior to be altered is stabilized. This is a minimum prerequisite for evaluating the effectiveness of interventive attempts.

In summary, all of these designs can be easily implemented in social work. Above all, they provide data which will enable a worker to determine if his/her interventions have had an effect on client behaviors (Wodarski & Buckholdt, 1975). It is not practicable to indicate what particular designs should be used at a given time, because this depends on the context of the social work practice situation, the behaviors to be modified, time considerations, administrative concerns, and so forth.[3]

Statistics

Evaluation will involve several means of assessing whether or not significant change has taken place. Evaluation of prevention services will entail the construction of tables and graphs of client and therapist behaviors. Usually, graphs are constructed from measures of central tendencies such as the mean, mode, or the median. A common error in social work practice is to focus solely on what is to be changed in the client and to proceed only to measure that. Sophisticated evaluation programs will measure the behaviors of the client and the change agent simultaneously in order to enable the assessment of what effects the change agent's behavior has had on the client. Guidelines regarding acceptable levels of change are being developed. They will indicate whether or not a program has had a positive effect in terms of the investment of professional effort, financial resources, and significance for the client (Gottman & Lieblum, 1974; Wodarski, Hudson, & Buckholdt, 1976). To aid in the evaluation endeavor, computer programs are now available that will summarize, graph, and place data in tabular form.[4]

Follow-Up

The proper assessment of any prevention program with children involves follow-up, a procedure employed by surprisingly few investigators. Crucial questions answered by follow-up include whether a prevention program has changed behaviors in a desired direction, how long these behaviors were maintained, and to what other contexts did they generalize. Pertinent questions remain as to when and where a follow-up should occur, for how long it should last, and who should secure the measurement. Consistent empirical guidelines for these are yet to be developed. It is posited that follow-up should occur for at least five years after the intervention to evaluate its effectiveness. Failure to provide an adequate follow-up period is a major deficiency of many evaluative studies executed in the social sciences.

Implementation of Findings

It is necessary for evaluators to relate their results to practitioners if social work practice knowledge is to be advanced. Formal and informal channels of communication can be employed to communicate the evaluation of therapeutic services. Formal channels may consist of professional newsletters, conferences, and journals. However, research indicates that these channels are not utilized frequently or that they do not influence practice behaviors as much as informal channels, e.g. indigenous leaders and peer relationships (Kolevzon, 1977; McNaul, 1972; Rosenblatt, 1968; Weed & Greenwald, 1973). Thus, the social work evaluator must assess indigenous leaders in the profession and determine what peer relationships influence practice behaviors most. They must then utilize these to communicate their research results and thereby influence practice.

SUMMARY

The establishment, implementation and evaluation of social work prevention programs for antisocial adolescents is an interrelated process. It has been emphasized that considerable time should be spent in dealing with the items reviewed here in order to establish a program which is relevant to client needs and which can be implemented in such a manner that enables a proper evaluation. Sufficient time spent in the planning and establishment phases greatly facilitates implementation and evaluation.

ENDNOTES

1. Such texts include Orval G. Johnson (Ed.), *Tests and measurements in child development: A handbook* (1976); and Paul McReynolds and Gordon Chelune (Eds.), *Advances in psychological assessment* (Vol. 6, 1984). Both are Jossey-Bass publications. Also see: Newmark, C. S. (Ed.), *Major psychological assessment instruments,* Rockleigh, NJ: Allyn and Bacon, Longwood Division, 1985; and Corcoran, K., and Fischer, J., *Measures for clinical practice: A sourcebook,* (New York: Free Press, 1987).

2. For an excellent discussion of measurement techniques see: Bijou, S. W., Peterson, R. F., Harris, F. R., Allen, K. E., & Johnston, M. W., "Methodology for experimental studies of young children in natural settings," *The Psychological Record,* 1969, *19*, 177-210; and Thomas, E. J. (Ed.), *Behavior modification procedure: A sourcebook,* (Chicago: Aldine, 1974).

3. For a detailed description of the various designs that might be used to evaluate social work practice interventions, see: Hersen, M., & Barlow, D. H., *Single case experimental designs* (1976); and Clifford J. Drew and Michael L. Hardman, *Designing and conducting behavioral research* (1986). Both are Pergamon publications.

4. The following computer program packages summarize, graph, and place data in tabular form: NYBMUL (Finn, J. D., Buffalo, NY: Computing Center Press, 1969); *SPSS* (Nie, N., Bent. D., & Hull, C. H., New York: McGraw-Hill, 1975); *BMD* (Dixon, W. J. (Ed.), Berkeley: University of California Press, 1970).

REFERENCES

Bandura, A. (1969). *Principles of behavior modification.* New York: Holt, Rinehart, and Winston.

Bandura, A. (1977). *Social learning theory.* Englewood Cliffs, NJ: Prentice-Hall.

Berkowitz, B. P., & Graziano, A. N. (1972). Training parents as behavior therapists: A review. *Behavior Research and Therapy, 10,* 297-317.

Bijou, S. W., Peterson, R. F., Harris, F. R., Allen, K. E., & Johnston, M. W. (1969). Methodology for experimental studies of young children in natural settings. *The Psychological Record, 19,* 177-210.

Brown, C. E. (Ed.). (1968). *The multi-problem dilemma.* Metuchen, NJ: The Scarecrow Press.

Carkhuff, R. R. (1969). *Helping and human relations.* New York: Holt, Rinehart, and Winston.

Carkhuff, R. R. (1971). Training as a preferred mode of treatment. *Journal of Counseling Psychology, 18,* 123-131.

Carkhuff, R. R., & Berenson, B. G. (1967). *Beyond counseling and therapy.* New York: Holt, Rinehart, and Winston.

Churchill, S. (1965). Social group work: A diagnostic tool in child guidance. *American Journal of Orthopsychiatry, 35,* 581-588.

Corrigan, J. O., Dell, D. M., Lewis, K.N., & Schmidt, L. E. (1980). Counseling as a social influence process: A review. *Journal of Counseling Psychology, 27*(4), 395-441.

Feldman, R. A., Caplinger, T. E., & Wodarski, J. S. (1983). *The St. Louis conundrum: The effective treatment of antisocial youths.* Englewood Cliffs, NJ: Prentice-Hall.

Fischer, J. (1973a). Has mighty casework struck out? *Social Work, 18*(4), 107-110.

Fischer, J. (1973b). Is casework effective? A review. *Social Work, 18*(11), 5-20.

Fischer, J. (1975). Training for effective therapeutic practice. *Psychotherapy, Research and Practice, 12*(1), 118-123.

Garfield, S. L. (1977). Research on the training of professional psychotherapists. In A. Gurman & A. Razin (Eds.), *Effective psychotherapy.* New York: Pergamon.

Geismar, L. L., LaGay, B., Wolock, I., Gerhart, V., & Fink, H. (1972). *Early support of family life.* Metuchen, NJ: Scarecrow Press.

Gottman, J. M., & Lieblum, S. R. (1974). *How to do psychotherapy and how to evaluate it.* New York: Holt, Rinehart, and Winston.

Gruver, G.G. (1971). College students as therapeutic agents. *Psychological Bulletin, 76*(2), 111-127.

Handler, E. (1975). Social work and corrections: Comments on an uneasy partnership. *Criminology, 13,* 240-254.

Henderson, R., & Shore, B. K. (1974). Accountability for what and to whom. *Social Work, 19*(4), 287-288.

Kazdin, A. E. (1975). *Behavior modification in applied settings.* Homewood, IL: Dorsey.

Kazdin, A. E. (1977). *The token economy.* New York: Plenum.

Kolevzon, M. (1977). Negative findings revisited: Implications for social work practice and education. *Clinical Social Work Journal, 5,* 210, 218.

Lipton, D., Martinson, R., & Wilks, J. (1975). *The effectiveness of correctional treatment: A survey of treatment evaluation studies.* New York: Praeger.

Lundman, R. J. (1976). Will diversion reduce recidivism? *Crime and Delinquency, 22*(4), 428-437.

Lundman, R. J., McFarlane, P. T., & Scarpitti, F. R. (1976). Delinquency prevention: Assessment of reported projects. *Crime and Delinquency, 22*(3), 297-308.

Meyer, H. J., Borgatta, E. F., & Jones, W. C. (1965). *Girls at vocational high: An experiment in social work intervention.* New York: Russell Sage Foundation.

McNaul, J. P. (1972). Relations between researchers and practitioners. In S. Z. Nagi & R. C. Corwin (Eds.), *The social contexts of research.* New York: Wiley.

Mullen, E. J., & Dumpson, J. R. (1972). *Evaluation of social intervention.* San Francisco: Jossey-Bass.

Nelson, R. O., Lipinski, D. P., & Black, J. L. (1975). The effects of expectancy on the reactivity of self-recording. *Behavior Therapy, 6*(3), 337-349.

Reid, J. W., & Shyne, A. W. (1969). *Brief and extended casework.* New York: Columbia University Press.

Rosenblatt, A. (1968). The practitioner's use and evaluation of research. *Social Work, 13*(1), 53-59.

Rosenthal, R. (1966). *Experimenter effects in behavioral research.* New York: Appleton-Century-Crofts.

Rosenthal, R., & Rosnow, R. L. (Eds.). (1969). *Artifact in behavioral research.* New York: Academic Press.

Sarri, R. C., & Selo, E. (1974). Evaluation process and outcome in juvenile correction: Musings on a grim tale. In P. Davidson, F. Clark, & L. Hammerlynck (Eds.), *Evaluation of behavioral programs in community, residential, and school settings.* Champaign, IL: Research Press.

Schinke, S. P., & Gilchrist, L. D. (1984). *Life skills counseling with adolescents.* Baltimore: University Park Press.

Schwartz, W. (1966). Neighborhood centers. In H. Maas (Ed.), *Five fields of social service: Reviews of research.* New York: National Association of Social Workers.

Schwartz, W. (1971). Neighborhood centers and group work. In H. Maas (Ed.), *Five fields of social service: Reviews of research.* New York: National Association of Social Workers.

Stokes, T. F., & Baer, D. M. (1977). An implicit technology of generalization. *Journal of Applied Behavior Analysis, 12*(2), 349-367.

Suinn, R. M. (1974). Traits for selection of paraprofessionals for behavior modification consultation training. *Community Mental Health Journal, 10*(4), 441-449.

Tharp, R. G., & Wetzel, R. J. (1969). *Behavior modification in the natural environment.* New York: Academic Press.

Truax, C. B., & Carkhuff, R. R. (1967). *Toward effective counseling and psychotherapy: Training and practice.* Chicago: Aldine-Atherton.

Vitalo, R. L. (1975). Guidelines in the functioning of a helping service. *Community Mental Health Journal, 11*(2), 170-178.

Voit, E. (1975). Social work and corrections: Another view. *Criminology, 13,* 255-270.

Weed, P., & Greenwald, S. R. (1973). The mystics of statistics. *Social Work, 18*(2), 113-115.

Wells, R. A., & Miller, D. (1973). Developing relationship skills in social work students. *Social Work Education Reporter, 21*(1), 60-73.

Wodarski, J. S. (1974). A behavioral program for the training of social group workers. *Journal of School Social Work, 1*(3), 38-54.

Wodarski, J. S. (1975). Use of videotapes in social work. *Clinical Social Work Journal, 3*(2), 120-127.

Wodarski, J. S. (1980). Legal requisites for social work practice. *Clinical Social Work Journal, 7*(4), 90-98.

Wodarski, J. S. (1985). An assessment model of practitioner skills: A prototype. *Arete, 10*(2), 1-14.

Wodarski, J. S. (1987). *Social work practice with children and adolescents.* Springfield, IL: Charles C Thomas.

Wodarski, J. S., & Buckholdt, D. (1975). Behavioral instruction in college classrooms: A review of methodological procedures. In J. Johnston (Ed.), *Behavior research and technology in higher education.* Springfield, IL: Charles C Thomas.

Wodarski, J. S., & Feldman, R. A. (1974). Practical aspects of field research. *Clinical Social Work Journal, 2*(3), 182-193.

Wodarski, J. S., Feldman, R. A., & Pedi, S. (1975). Labeling by self and others: The comparison of behavior among antisocial and prosocial children in an open community agency. *Criminal Justice and Behavior, 2*(3), 258-275.

Wodarski, J. S., Feldman, R. A., & Pedi, S. (1976a). The comparison of antisocial and prosocial children on multicriterion measures at summer camp. *Journal of Abnormal Child Psychology, 3*(3), 255-273.

Wodarski, J. S., Feldman, R. A., & Pedi, S. (1976b). The comparison of antisocial and prosocial children on multicriterion measures at summer camp: A three-year study. *Social Service Review, 50*(2), 256-272.

Wodarski, J. S., Hudson, W., & Buckholdt, D. (1976). Issues in evaluative research: Implications for social work. *Journal of Sociology and Social Welfare, 4*(1), 81-113.

Wodarski, J. S., & Pedi, S. (1977). The comparison of antisocial and prosocial children on multicriterion measures at a community center: A three year study. *Social Work, 22,* 290-296.

Wodarski, J. S., Pippin, J., & Daniels, M. (1988). Effects of graduate social work education on personality, values, and interpersonal skills. *Journal of Social Work Education, 24*(3), 266-277.

Chapter 3

CURRICULUMS AND PRACTICAL ASPECTS
OF IMPLEMENTATION

PREVENTION ENDEAVORS should occur in the fourth, fifth, or
sixth grades. These grades are appropriate because they are pre-
adolescent years. Adolescents should be equipped with knowledge in the
areas of sexuality, substance abuse, and so forth. Also, an appropriate
rationale for these areas is that these are the years that the adolescent
needs to be equipped with specific knowledge to deal with peer influences that will occur on cognitive and social behaviors. In order to
successfully accomplish the developmental tasks of adolescence, i.e.
transition from adolescence to adulthood, teens need a structured, stable, and moderately restrained environment.

Accumulated data indicate that adolescents who are at risk possess
the following characteristics: those who have high family instability,
such as high level of conflict between spouses and their adolescents;
low economic status; lack of religious affiliation; lack of church attendance; lack of appropriate parental management of the adolescent;
lack of social connections with peers; and low grades (Ek & Steelman,
1988).

MODELS OF SERVICE

There are two means to deliver services to adolescents — the implementation of the programs in semistructured contexts and the use of
more structured peer learning structures through the use of the Teams-
Games-Tournaments (TGT) technique.

Social Skills Training: Semistructured Approach

The social skills preparation approach is based on an amalgamation of Goldstein and his colleagues' (1980) structured learning model, "Skill-streaming the Adolescent"; Gazda's (1982) life span development skills adolescent program; and Gurney's (1977) relationship enhancement model. The emphasis is on imparting transferable social skills-attitudes.

Social skills may be thought of as overt (verbal and non-verbal components of overt social behaviors) and covert (internal skills affecting self-control and problem-solving abilities across all social settings and circumstances) learned behaviors that maximize chances for obtaining positive reinforcement from social interactions while minimizing cost to self and others (Gilchrist, 1981).

Social skills training typically consists of the following components: (1) a rationale as to why a given social behavior is desirable; (2) an opportunity to observe examples of the behavior (i.e. modeling); (3) an opportunity to practice the behavior, usually in role-play situations; and (4) corrective feedback regarding performance (Rusch, 1986).

Research indicates that it is necessary to teach youths at risk social skills and attitudes necessary for them to successfully develop relevant educational competencies; handle current problems and stresses; anticipate and prevent future problems; and advance their mental health, social functioning, and economic welfare. Initially, adolescents' social skills-attitudes should be assessed. Subsequently, they should participate in a series of psychoeducational "courses," including vocational enrichment (Azrin, 1978), enhancing interpersonal relationships (Lange & Jakubowski, 1976), managing stress and building social responsibility (Schinke & Gilchrist, 1984), determining alternatives to aggression and dealing with feelings (Goldstein, Sprafkin, Gershaw, & Klein, 1980), and problem solving (D'Zurilla & Goldfried, 1971; Spivack & Shure, 1974).

A variety of psychoeducational methods are employed in the "courses," including individual and group counseling, self-assessments, live and videotape demonstrations, behavioral rehearsal with counselor, peer and videotape feedback, written materials, positive reinforcement, individual and group contracts, buddy systems, and progress logs. Most of these therapeutic strategies are delivered through a group work approach (Feldman & Wodarski, 1975; Wodarski, 1981).

The Group Context for Training

Even though recent years have witnessed a growing emphasis on group treatment, relatively few youths at risk are treated in this manner.

The provision of services in groups offers the following positive aspects. The group interactional situation more frequently typifies many kinds of daily interactions. Services that facilitate the development of behaviors which enable people to interact in groups are likely to better prepare them for participation in larger society; that is, will help them learn social skills necessary to secure reinforcement (Feldman & Wodarski, 1975; Wodarski, 1981). From a social learning theory perspective, it is posited that if a behavior is learned in a group context, it is likely to come under the control of a greater number of discriminative stimuli; therefore, greater generalization of the behavior can occur for a broader variety of interactional contexts.

The group context of the various skills programs is intended to capitalize on the adolescent's dependence on peers. Group identity and cohesion should be fostered within groups of adolescents. Group support can be mobilized to aid individuals at moments of particular difficulty (Ross & Glaser, 1973). The group interaction situation typifies many kinds of daily living situations, and the group provides a context where new behaviors can be tested in a realistic atmosphere (Feldman & Wodarski, 1975).

There are additional substantiated rationales for working with individuals in groups. Groups provide a context where new behaviors can be tested in a realistic atmosphere. Adolescents can get immediate peer feedback and support regarding their problem-solving behaviors. They are provided with role models to facilitate the acquisition of requisite social behavior. Groups provide a more valid focus for accurate diagnosis and a more potent means for changing client behavior (Meyer & Smith, 1977; Rose, 1977; Wodarski, 1981).

Lack of interpersonal relationship skills plays a significant role in the youth's inability to attain and maintain educational success and in their general dissatisfaction with life. Services structured in a group manner should help these individuals practice necessary social skills to facilitate their acquisition, thus enhancing their interpersonal relationships and educational opportunities. Additionally, many youth at risk feel emptiness, social isolation and a sense of failure and could benefit from the support derived from the group. Finally, the provision of services through groups greatly increases the number of clients who can be served by an effective treatment program (Wodarski & Bagarozzi, 1979).

The Teams-Games-Tournaments Technique

The use of small team learning groups over the last fifteen years has been applied to the solution of many classroom problems, including discipline and the teaching of verbal, reading and arithmetic skills. These are the first curriculums developed to teach knowledge and social skills to secondary students through small group learning procedures.

The Teams-Games-Tournaments (TGT) technique was developed through extensive research on games as teaching devices, on small groups as classroom work units, and on task and reward structures used in the traditional classroom. TGT has a successful history with traditionally hard subjects to teach, such as nutrition, social studies, and so forth. TGT is an alternate teaching mechanism which fully utilizes a reward structure that emphasizes group rather than individual achievement (Feldman & Wodarski, 1975; Wodarski, Adelson, Tidball, & Wodarski, 1980; Wodarski, 1981). This is preferred over individual classroom instruction education for several reasons. First, the group learning situation most closely resembles the setting in which adolescents make their decisions regarding high-risk behaviors among peers. And since high-risk behaviors most often take place in group settings, knowledge acquired in the group setting is more likely to be used when in similar peer group settings than knowledge acquired through individual, separate means (Allman, Taylor & Nathan, 1972; Feldman & Wodarski, 1975; Wodarski & Bagarozzi, 1979). From the perspective of the educator, the group method allows for a broader range of learning experience; students have the opportunity to learn while interacting with peers in a friendly, exciting game.

The special timeliness of TGT to teach adolescents about high-risk behaviors and how to make better decisions regarding its usage is that when TGT is used, all students have an equal opportunity to succeed, because all students compete against members of other teams who are at similar achievement levels, and points earned by low achievers are just as valuable to the overall team score as points earned by high achievers.

The three basic elements in this technique which promote motivation and interest in learning are teams, games, and tournaments.

Teams. Before beginning the education phase of the program, students are assessed for level of knowledge of high-risk behaviors. The completion of the pretest of knowledge provides the basis for division of students in four-member teams. The teams are organized into high achievers (those with a high level of knowledge of high-risk behaviors), middle achievers (those with moderate levels), and low achievers (those most lacking in knowledge of high-risk behaviors). Team composition is heterogenous, with one high achiever, two middle achievers, and one low achiever on each team, so that the average achievement level is approximately equal across teams. The team remains intact throughout the period when TGT is used. The day before a tournament, team members hold a team practice session to study together or to fill out worksheets reviewing the material covered that week. Peer tutoring is encouraged.

Games. Students compete against members of other teams on instructional games which are provided in the curriculum guide. The games are usually short-answer questions designed to assess and reinforce the material taught in class.

Tournaments. Students play the games in tournaments held weekly. Each student is assigned to a tournament table where he/she competes individually against two other students, each representing a different team. The students at each table are of comparable achievement levels. Points are earned for each game question answered correctly, and at the end of the tournament, the top, middle and low scorers get a fixed number of points. Each player receives some points for participating in the tournament. The points a student earns are used to determine whether he/she will be "bumped" to the next higher table (with high performing students), "bumped" to the next lower table, or stay at the same table for the next tournament. This bumping procedure encourages students who have increased their achievement levels to keep working. The points are added to those earned by other members of the student's team to compute a team score. The individual and team scores should be ranked and publicized in a tournament newsletter for the class.

The education units centering on high-risk behaviors provided in various guides are to be presented for fifty minutes each day for four to six weeks. The first three days of each week are to be devoted to learning high-risk behaviors and concepts in the exercises, discussions and various participatory activities. The fourth day is to be focused on working in the TGT teams on worksheets in preparation for the tournament which is to be held on the fifth day of each week.

CURRICULUMS AVAILABLE

Components of Each Model

Each intervention package must have attractive and effective means of practicing behaviors. A requisite component of each intervention is a presentation of essential knowledge and development of requisite skills in the implementation of the knowledge.

Sex Education

The Comprehensive Sexual Education Program is designed to provide early adolescents with basic physiological knowledge about both sexes, as well as certain basic values concerning sexuality. This is done by means of parental communication and peer group experience within the school, thus increasing the likelihood that the adolescent will have an enjoyable learning experience and an opportunity to strengthen the relationship with his/her parent(s). The program is two-tiered. Adolescents focus educationally on human reproductive physiology, gender and role enhancement, peer skills development, and problem solving. Parents focus on human productive physiology, communication skills with adolescents, values clarification, and the relational aspects of sexuality.

Substance Abuse

The Comprehensive Psychoactive Substance Use Education Program for Adolescents is targeted to provide essential knowledge to adolescents about psychoactive substances in such a manner as to be a fun, peer group experience, thus increasing the likelihood of acquisition of knowledge and behavior. The program is comprised of three parts: education about psychoactive substances, self-management skills related to substance use, and the maintenance of knowledge and behavior.

The instructional method of the comprehensive program is the Teams-Games-Tournaments (TGT) technique. The TGT technique is an innovative teaching technique which has been used extensively in the past to teach science, mathematics, and nutrition. The special timeliness of the TGT technique to teach adolescents about psychoactive substances is that it utilizes a group rather than an individual reward structure. This is preferable with adolescents for several reasons. First, the group learning situation most closely resembles the setting in which adolescents make their decisions regarding the use of psychoactive substances—amongst peers. Teaching procedures which facilitate the level of knowledge needed to make healthy decisions are likely to better prepare adolescents to use that knowledge when in the group setting in their normal environment where using decisions take place. The group setting is conducive to the production of role models to identify with for lower achieving youth, and allows for a broader range of learning experiences other than strictly paper-and-pencil methods with little incorporation of others' experiences. In addition, the peer involvement and support network development by the small group method will greatly enhance the acquisition of knowledge.

Adolescent Depression and Suicide

Research has established the association between suicidal behavior in adolescents and depressive symptoms. A chronic inability to cope with changing life situations has been identified as a major factor in depression and as a predictor in suicidal attempts. This manual provides a guide for an intervention treatment for combatting adolescent depression and subsequent suicide. It is proposed for use by psychotherapists practicing in hospitals and outpatient clinics.

Treatment of suicidal adolescents requires using all available methods and resources separately, sequentially, and in conjunction. This treatment manual offers basic training to help adolescents identify a potential suicide and respond effectively. This manual includes four treatment components: information about depression and suicide; self-management skills related to depression with the following foci: problem solving, increasing interpersonal skills, and stress reduction through relaxation; social and family interactional skills; and the maintenance of knowledge and behavior.

Of vital importance to a treatment program is the teaching of skills adolescents need in order to cope with the stresses of everyday life. Numerous studies have connected suicidal behavior to depression, stress, family disruption, and poor peer relationships. This intervention is targeted to provide essential knowledge and skills to adolescents for depression management and suicide prevention. The program utilizes a peer group experience to increase the likelihood of acquisition and maintenance of knowledge and behavior.

Employment Preparation

This curriculum presents a comprehensive employment preparation intervention for adolescents with developmental disabilities. Vocational preparation is viewed in terms of the development of job skills and related psychosocial skills.

The Comprehensive Employment Preparation Program is designed as a means of helping youth and young adults with developmental disabilities acquire skills necessary to prepare them for effective functioning as self-sustaining, *working* members of society. Substantial research indicates that the lack of social, problem-solving and employment-seeking skills is a significant factor in attaining and maintaining employment. At this time, relevant educational and psychological literature clearly reveals progress is being made in our ability to appropriately assess individual deficiencies and program for development of improved social competency, i.e. problem-solving, interpersonal and vocational competencies.

Violent Children: A Prevention Paradigm

The intervention has early identification and intervention based on empirical knowledge with youths exhibiting high rates of antisocial behavior. Parents are taught adequate parenting skills, with emphasis on communication. This approach alleviates the deleterious circumstances that affect potentially violent children. These children can be identified by an inflated rate of antisocial behavior or through contact with the law. Children are taught life skills in the following areas: cognitive anger control, problem solving, peer enhancement, and substance abuse education (Spence & Marzillier, 1981; Kaplan, Konecni, & Novaco, 1984). By introducing interventions at both home and school, it can be determined which is most effective, either singularly or in combination, in helping aggressive youngsters overcome their antisocial tendencies.

ASSESSMENT MEASURES

The following section contains those measures that we have found helpful in our research. We have chosen them based on the criteria of having adequate realiability and ease of administration in this time of energy and costs.

Sex Knowledge

Sex Knowledge Test (Kirby, 1984)

This inventory is a 34-item, multiple-choice scale. It includes questions in the following areas: adolescent physical development, adolescent relationships, adolescent sexual activity, adolescent pregnancy, adolescent marriage, the probability of pregnancy, birth control, and sexually transmitted disease. The test was developed after literature and overall goals of sexuality education were examined. The test-retest reliability of the knowledge test was determined by administering the test to 58 adolescents on two occasions, two weeks apart, and then calculating the correlation coefficient between their total score on the first administration and their total score on the second administration. The reliability coefficient is .89.

Behavior Inventory (Kirby, 1984)

Three aspects of behaviors were considered in developing these measures. These are the skill with which the behavior is completed, the comfort experienced during that behavior, and the frequency of that behavior. The Behavior Inventory measures these three aspects in:

(1) skills in taking responsibility for personal behavior
(2) social decision-making skills
(3) sexual decision making
(4) communication skills
(5) assertiveness skills
(6) birth control assertiveness skills
(7) comfort engaging in social activities
(8) comfort talking about sex and birth control
(9) comfort expressing concern and caring
(10) comfort being assertive sexually
(11) comfort having current sex life
(12) comfort getting and using birth control
(13) existence and frequency of sexual activity
(14) frequency of use of birth control
(15) frequency of communication about sex and birth control with parents
(16) frequency of communication about sex and birth control with friends
(17) frequency of communication about sex and birth control with boy/girlfriend.

The questions measuring skills use five-point scales; the questions measuring comfort use four-point Likert-type scales; while the questions measuring sexual activity, use of birth control, and frequency of communication ask how many times during the previous month the respondent engaged in the specific activity.

Test-retest coefficients indicate that the items have a great range of reliability coefficients. The scales measuring skills range from poor (.57) to excellent (.88). Scales measuring comfort range from a low of .38 (comfort getting and using birth control) to a high of .70 (comfort having current sex life). The questions involving sexual activity had excellent reliability. The questions about whether or not respondents have ever had intercourse had a reliability of 1.00. The items measuring frequencies of communication have an adequate, but not excellent, reliability (Kirby, 1984).

Attitude and Values Inventory (Kirby, 1984)

This instrument includes 15 different scales, each consisting of five-point Likert-type items measuring the following:

   (1) clarity of long-term goals
   (2) clarity of personal sexual values
   (3) understanding of personal sexual values
   (4) understanding of emotional needs
   (5) understanding of personal social behavior
   (6) understanding of personal sexual responses
   (7) attitudes toward various gender role behaviors
   (8) attitudes toward sexuality in life
   (9) attitudes toward the importance of birth control
  (10) attitudes toward premarital intercourse
  (11) attitudes toward the use of pressure and force in sexual activity
  (12) recognition of the importance of the family
  (13) self-esteem
  (14) satisfaction with personal sexuality
  (15) satisfaction with social relationships

The reliability of the fifteen different scales was determined two different ways. First, the test-retest reliabilities were found by administering the questionnaire twice, two weeks apart, to 51 participants in different programs and then calculating the correlation coefficient between the first administration and the second administration of each scale. Second, the overall reliability of each scale was calculated by randomly selecting about 100 pretest and posttest questionnaires from each site, combining the questionnaires into a single file, and then calculating Cronbach's alpha for the items in each scale. Basically, using all of these measures of reliability, scales of clarity of goals and values range from a coefficient of .54 to .90; scales addressing understanding of needs, social behavior and response range from .51 to .84; attitude scales range from .30 to .94; self-esteem scales range from .73 to .80; and satisfaction scales range from .64 to .88.

Instructional Evaluation for Students (Kirby, 1984)

This class evaluation contains two parts. The first part asks the respondents to rate numerous teaching skills of the instructor, characteristics of classroom interaction, and program structure and materials. The second part asks participants to assess as accurately as possible the current or future effects of the course. In particular, it asks how the course affected their:

(1) knowledge
(2) understanding of personal behavior
(3) clarity of values
(4) attitude toward birth control
(5) communication about sexuality
(6) communication with parents
(7) probability of having sex

Anger Inventory (Novaco, 1975)

This is a 90-item instrument that presents hypothetical anger-evoking situations. Responses are made on a 5-point Likert scale indicating degree of anger.

Jesness Inventory (Jesness, 1969)

A personality inventory specifically designed for youth between ages 8 and 18, the Jesness Inventory is a brief (155-item) true-false questionnaire with easily comprehended, idiomatic items yielding 10 trait scores and a powerful index predictive of asocial tendencies. The inventory has also been used successfully with adults.

Scales are: Social Maladjustment, Value Orientation, Immaturity, Autism, Alienation, Manifest Aggression, Withdrawal, Social Anxiety, Repression, Denial, and the Asocial Index. Three scales and the Index were developed against external criteria, the others by cluster analysis (Tyron). Norms are based on delinquent and non-delinquent boys and girls with special attention to the inclusion of subjects from lower-middle and lower socioeconomic levels.

Psychoactive Substance Dependent Variables

Students' Knowledge About Drugs

An inventory will be prepared from the curriculum guide for pretest and posttest purposes. Each will contain 100 items randomly chosen from a pool of 200 for the pre and posttest.

Thirty-six items from the Engs Inventory will assess knowledge about alcohol (Engs, 1977a, 1977b; Engs, Decoster, Larson, & McPherson, 1978). This inventory has adequate reliability and validity.

The Drug Educational Scales consist of 41 multiple-choice items of five types of commonly abused drugs: marijuana, hallucinogens, stimulants, depressants, and opiates (Horan & Williams, 1975). For sufficient reliability, the inventory will have been updated for the proposed project.

Self-Inventories

The self-inventory is designed to measure current drug use and any current problem drug behavior, students' attitudes and intentions about drug use, motivation, and peer influence to experiment with drugs.

Self-reports of drinking behavior are measured by 23 items of the Engs Inventory (Engs, 1977a, 1977b).

Drug Use Behavior Questionnaire. Items center on drug use behavior (28 items); psychosocial aspects of drug use (6 items); adverse reactions to marijuana usage (7 items); psychological health (11 items); SES and economics (8 items); deviance (6 items); accidents and hospitalization (5 items); physical health (17 items); leisure time (9 items); interpersonal relations (8 items); life satisfaction (24 items); short-term or immediate drug effects (10 items); and long-term effects (16 items) (Lettieri, 1981). Substantial reliability and validity are available on quality and relevance of the items.

Smart Questionnaire includes measures of cigarette smoking, alcohol use, marijuana use, and intentions to use tobacco, alcohol, and marijuana, as well as measures of numerous psychosocial constructs. Extensive reliability indicates acceptable range (Graham, Flay, Johnson, Hansen, Grossman, & Sobel, 1984).

Conflict Behavior Questionnaire (CBQ)

The CBQ (Prinz, Foster, Kent, & O'Leary, 1979) consists of 75 (parent form) or 73 (adolescent form) items measuring perceived conflict of behavior at home. Family conflict is perceived to be marked by disapproval of and complaints about the behavior of the other. On the CBQ, parents and adolescents independently complete yes-no ratings of items on two potential sources of complaints: general dissatisfaction with the other person's behavior and evaluations of the interactions between the two members. Two scores are computed with higher scores representing the number of negatively endorsed items describing the other's behavior (individual scale — CBQ-Ind.) and describing the dyadic interaction (dyadic scale — CBQ-Dyad). Adequate reliability and validity are available (Prinz et al., 1979; Robin & Foster, 1984; Robin & Weiss, 1980).

Issues Checklist (IC)

The IC (Prinz et al., 1979) is an instrument designed to assess the occurrence, frequency, and intensity of discussions of particular issues that may arise between parent and adolescent. The IC includes 44 issues that represent potential concern for parents and adolescents. Representative issues are fighting with brothers and sisters, use of the telephone, drug use, and how to spend free time. The checklist is completed independently by each parent and the adolescent. For each issue, the respondent is asked to identify: (1) whether the issue had been discussed during the last four weeks (yes or no); (2) if yes, how many times in the last month it had been discussed; and (3) when it was discussed, how angry or intense the discussions were (rated on a 5-point scales from 1 = calm to 5 = angry.

When averaged across issues one can obtain a summary score or quantity of issues discussd, mean frequency of discussion per issue, mean anger-intensity level, and a weighted average of the frequency and anger-intensity level of the endorsed issues. Prinz et al. (1979) and Robin and Weiss (1980) provide reliability and validity data for this measure.

Conflict Perception Ratings

This measure will be utilized to assess individuals' perceptions and conflict (poor communication) in objective dyadic interactions. Scenes are based on work by Smith and Forehand (in press). Themes for the scenes were chosen from the Issues Checklist (Prinz et al., 1979). Themes for the present project will be two scenes representing a low level of conflict between adolescents and parents, two scenes representing a moderate level of conflict, and two scenes representing a high level of conflict between parents and adolescents. For each level of conflict, one scene will consist of a mother-adolescent interaction and one will consist of a father-adolescent interaction. Twenty scenes were read by pairs of actors and were recorded on audiotapes. These tapes were then rated by observers who had been trained in the rating of conflict and communication. Each observer rated each tape on a 7-point Likert scale assessing the amount of conflict in the interaction. Based on the ratings conducted by these observers, scenes that fit into low (rating of 1), medium (rating of 4), and high (rating of 7) levels of conflict were selected.

Subjects will listen to the six audiotaped scenes (which will be presented in a random order) and will score each interaction on a 7-point Likert scale (1 indicating little conflict and 7 indicating high conflict).

Parent Measures

(1) Parents' knowledge about drugs (will be a modified version of the two adolescent drug knowledge measures).

(2) Self-inventories designed to measure current drug use, any current problem drug behavior, attitudes and intentions about drug use, and motivation (see adolescent measures above).

(3) Knowledge of Social Learning Principles (O'Dell, Tarler-Benlolo, & Flynn, 1977). This instrument will be administered to assess parental understanding of basic social learning principles as they apply to children/adolescents. The KBPAC is a 45-item, multiple-choice instrument that has been used in prior research and has been shown to adequately reflect changes in parental knowledge in social learning principles (McMahon, Forehand, & Griest, 1981).

(4) Conflict Behavior Questionnaire (see adolescent measures above)

(5) Issues Checklist (see adolescent measures above)

(6) Conflict Communication Perception Ratings (see adolescent measures above)

(7) Revised Behavior Problem Checklist (RBPC). This instrument (Quay & Peterson, 1983) will be used to assess parent perceptions of adolescent deviance. Based on extensive analyses, four major factors have emerged from the RBPC: (a) conduct disorder, (b) socialized aggression, (c) attention problem-immaturity, and (d) anxiety-withdrawal. The factors of the 77-item scale were derived from factor analytic studies, and intercorrelation among the factors has been minimized by retaining those items that loaded highly on only one factor. Data that have been gathered on inpatient and outpatient psychiatric populations and normal samples suggest that the RBPC and its factors have adequate reliability and validity (Quay & Peterson, 1983).

Depression

Knowledge of Depression and Suicide

This scale assesses adolescents' knowledge of depression and suicide (questions drawn from educational material and information provided during the program intervention).

Self-Reports of Depression

Beck Depression Inventory. One of the most widely used measures in assessing the outcomes of depression. The inventory consists of 22 items with four to six responses per item (Lewinsohn et al., 1984).

Reynolds Adolescent Depression Scale. The RADS, developed to assess depressive symptomatology in adolescents, consists of 30 items reflecting DSM (American Psychiatric Association, 1980) symptomatology for major and minor (i.e. dysthymia) depression. Reynolds (1985, 1986), in studies with over 8,000 adolescents, has shown the RADS to be a reliable ($r = .92$ to $.96$, $r = .80$) and valid ($r = .71$ to $.83$ with self-report and clinical interview scales of depression) measure of depression in adolescents.

The Measurement of Depression. A self-rating scale (SDS) for the quantitative measurement of depression as an emotional disorder. The SDS is comprised of a list of 20 items. Each relates to a specific characteristic of depression (Zung, 1974).

Generalized Contentment Scale. This 25-item scale, rated on a 1-5 continuum, is designed to measure the degree, severity, or magnitude of nonpsychotic depression (Hudson, 1982).

Index of Self-Esteem. This 25-item scale, rated on a 1-5 continuum, is designed to measure the degree, severity, or magnitude of a client's problem with self-esteem, i.e. how he/she perceives him/herself (Hudson, 1982).

Manifest Alienation. This 20-item measure, rated on a 3-point continuum, is designed to determine the existence of an alienation syndrome in an individual. Alienation syndrome consists of feelings of pessimism, cynicism, distrust, apathy, and emotional distance (Gould, 1969).

Instruments Assessing Family Function

Index of Family Relations. This index is designed to measure the degree, severity, or magnitude of a problem as felt or perceived by the client that pertains to relationships of family members to one another. It can be regarded as a measure of intrafamilial stress and as a measure of the client's family environment (Hudson, Acklin, & Bartosh, 1980).

Child's Attitude Toward Mother. This index is designed to measure the degree, severity, or magnitude of a problem a child has with his/her mother (Giuli & Hudson, 1977).

Child's Attitude Toward Father. This index is designed to measure the degree, severity, or magnitude of a problem a child has with his/her father (Giuli & Hudson, 1977).

Parental Attitude Scale. This index is designed to measure the degree, severity, or magnitude of a problem a parent has in a relationship with his/her child or children, regardless of the age of the child (Hudson, Wung, & Borges, 1980).

Quality of Life. An adolescent form (25 items) and a parent form (40 items) are available. The adolescent form rates satisfaction on a 1-5 continuum for the following areas: family life, friends, extended family, health, home, education, leisure, religion, mass media, financial well-being, and neighborhood and community. The parent form rates satisfaction on a 1-5 continuum for the following areas: marriage and family life, friends, extended family, health, home, education, time, religion, employment, mass media, financial well-being, and neighborhood and community (Olson, McCubbin, Barnes, Larsen, Muxen, & Wilson, 1982).

Conflict Behavior Questionnaire (CBQ). The CBQ (Prinz et al., 1979) consists of 75 (parent form) or 73 (adolescent form) items measuring perceived conflict of behavior at home. Family conflict is perceived to be marked by disapproval of and complaints about the behavior of the other. On the CBQ, parents and adolescents independently complete yes-no ratings of items on two potential sources of complaints: general dissatisfaction with the other person's behavior and evaluations of the interactions between the two members. Two scores are computed, with higher scores representing the number of negatively endorsed items describing the other's behavior (individual scale—CBQ-Ind.) and describing dyadic interaction (dyadic scale—CBQ-Dyad). Adequate reliability and validity are available (Prinz et al., 1979; Robin & Foster, 1984; Robin & Weiss, 1980). Both adolescents and parents will complete this questionnaire.

Issues Checklist (IC). The IC (Prinz et al., 1979) is an instrument designed to assess the occurrence, frequency, and intensity of discussions of particular issues that may arise between parent and adolescent. The IC includes 44 issues that represent potential concern for parents and adolescents. Representative issues are fighting with brothers and sisters, use of the telephone, drug use, and how to spend free time. The checklist is independently completed by each parent and the adolescent. For each issue, the respondent is asked to identify: (1) whether the issue had been discussed during the last four weeks (yes or no); (2) if yes, how many times in the last month it had been discussed; and (3) when it was discussed, how angry or intense the discussions were (rated on a 5-point scale from 1 = calm to 5 = angry.

When averaged across issues one can obtain a summary score for quantity of issues discussed, mean frequency of discussion per issue, mean anger-intensity level, and a weighted average of the frequency and anger-intensity level of the endorsed issues. The last measure will be utilized in this study. It should be noted that Prinz et al. (1979) and Robin and Weiss (1980) provide reliability and validity data for this measure. Both adolescents and parents will complete this measure.

Conflict Perception Ratings. This measure will be utilized to assess individuals' perceptions of conflict (poor communication) in objective dyadic interactions. Scenes are based on work by Smith and Forehand (in press). Themes for the scenes where chosen from the Issues Checklist (Prinz et al., 1979). Themes for the present project will be two scenes representing a low level of conflict between adolescents and parents, two scenes representing a moderate level of conflict, and two scenes representing a high level of conflict between parents and adolescents. For each level of conflict, one scene will consist of a mother-adolescent interaction and one will consist of a father-adolescent interaction. Twenty scenes were read by pairs of actors and were recorded on audiotapes. These tapes were then rated by observers who had been trained in the rating of conflict and communication. Each observer rated each tape on a 7-point Likert scale assessing the amount of conflict in the interaction. Based on the ratings conducted by these observers, scenes that fit into low (rating of 1), medium (rating of 4), and high (rating of 7) levels of conflict were selected.

Subjects will listen to the six audiotaped scenes (which will be presented in a random order) and will score each interaction on a 7-point Likert scale (1 indicating little conflict and 7 indicating high conflict). Both adolescents and parents will complete this measure.

Knowledge of Social Learning Principles. This instrument (O'Dell, Tarler-Benlolo, & Flynn, 1977) will be administered to assess parental understanding of basic social learning principles as they apply to children/adolescents. The KBPAC is a 45-item, multiple-choice instrument that has been used in prior research and has been shown to adequately reflect changes in parental knowledge in social learning principles (McMahon, Forehand, & Griest, 1981). Parents complete this questionnaire.

Inventories Assessing Life Skills: Stress

State-Trait Anxiety Inventory. The STAI is the most widely used measure of anxiety throughout the world. It consists of two 20-item self-report scales designed to assess anxiety-proneness (trait) and current level of anxiety (state) (Spielberger, 1983).

A-File. This inventory consists of 50 items designed to record normative and non-normative life events and changes adolescents perceive their families have experienced during the past 12 months. The 50 items center on role of status transitions, sexuality, family losses, responsibilities and strains, school strains, and substance use and legal conflicts (Olson et al., 1982).

Inventories Assessing Life Skills: Problem Solving

The Social Means-Ends Problem-Solving Procedure (MEPS). The MEPS for adolescents was developed by Platt et al. (1974) to assess means-ends thinking in 13-18-year-olds. The measure consists of four stories that ask the subject to provide the means by which the character in the story arrives at a given end. All stories are of an interpersonal nature. Scores on the MEPS are arrived at by totaling the number of means stated toward a given story goal and the number of obstacles that might be encountered on the way to that goal (Platt & Spivack, 1975).

Emotional Means-Ends Problem-Solving Procedure (EMPS). The EMPS is a variation of the MEPS which asks for problem solving of negative emotional situations such as relieving oneself from depression and overcoming anxiety. Siegel et al. (1976) developed four story situations to measure this aspect of problem-solving ability in adolescents and adults. The EMPS is administered and scored in the same manner as the social MEPS.

Inventories Assessing Life Skills: Assertiveness

Assertive Inventory. A widely used inventory consisting of 40 items, rated on a 5-point scale (Gambrill & Richey, 1975).

Inventories Assessing Life Skills: Peer Relations

Index of Peer Relations. This 25-item scale, rated on a 1-5 continuum, is designed to measure the degree, severity, or magnitude of a client's problem in relationships with peers. It can be used as a global measure of peer relationship problems, or the therapist can specify the peer reference group (i.e. work associates, friends, classmates) (Hudson, 1982).

Behavioral Measurement

Living in Familial Environments (LIFE) Coding System. The LIFE Coding System was developed for the study of the interactions of depressed women and their families (Arthur, Hops, & Biglan, 1982). This will be altered appropriately to assess the adolescents in three two-hour sessions in the first, fourth and sixth weeks of intervention. The coding system was adopted from the Family Interaction Coding System (FICS: Reid, 1978) and the Marital Interaction Coding System (MICS: Hops, Willis, Patterson, & Weiss, 1972). The major modification involved the addition of content codes which were felt to be characteristic of depressed people and the addition of seven codes for affective behavior. The coding system contained 31 content and 7 affect categories. For the purposes of the present study, these categories were collapsed on a prior basis into seven categories: (1) depressive, (2) aggressive, (3) facilitative, (4) solution proposal, (5) self-disclosure, (6) elicit response, and (7) other.

SUMMARY

This chapter has elaborated the curriculums available. The programs equip adolescents with the necessary knowledge and relevant social skills to avoid and neutralize risk situations. Each curriculum has a corresponding family component to support the education and skills aspects of the prevention intervention. Lastly, relevant assessment procedures have been elaborated.

REFERENCES

Allman, R., Taylor, H. A., & Nathan, P. E. (1972). Group drinking during stress: Effects on drinking behavior, affect and psychopathology. *American Journal of Psychiatry, 129*(6), 45-54.

American Psychiatric Association. (1980). *Diagnostic and statistical manual of mental disorders* (3rd ed.). Washington, DC: Author.

Arthur, J. A., Hops, H., & Biglan, A. (1982). *LIFE (living in familial environments) coding system.* Unpublished manuscript, Oregon Research Institute, Eugene, OR.

Azrin, N. H., (1978, November). *A learning approach to job finding.* Paper presented at the Association for Advancement of Behavior Therapy, Chicago.

D'Zurilla, T. J., & Goldfried, M. R. (1971). Problem solving and behavior modification. *Journal of Abnormal Psychology, 78,* 101-126.

Ek, C. A., & Steelman, L. C. (1988). Becoming a runaway: From the accounts of youthful runners. *Youth & Society, 19*(3), 334-358.

Engs, R. C. (1977a). Drinking patterns and drinking problems of college students. *Journal of Studies on Alcohol, 38*(11), 2144-2156.

Engs, R. C. (1977b). Let's look before we leap: The cognitive and behavioral evaluation of a university alcohol education program. *Journal of Alcohol and Drug Education, 22*(2).

Engs, R. C., Decoster, D., Larson, R. V., & McPherson, P. (1978). The drinking behavior of college students and cognitive effects of a voluntary alcohol education program. *National Association of Student Personnel Administration, 15*(3), 59-64.

Feldman, R. A., & Wodarski, J. S. (1975). *Contemporary approaches to group treatment.* San Francisco: Jossey-Bass.

Gambrill, E. D., & Richey, C. A. (1975). An assertion inventory for use in assessment and research. *Behavior Therapy, 6,* 550-561.

Gazda, G. M. (1982). Life skills training. In E. Marchall & D. Kurtz (Eds.), *Interpersonal helping skills.* San Francisco: Jossey-Bass.

Gilchrist, L. D. (1981). Social competence in adolescence. In S. Schinke (Ed.), *Behavioral methods in social welfare* (pp. 61-80). New York: Aldine.

Giuli, C. A., & Hudson, W. W. (1977). Assessing parent-child relationship disorders in clinical practice: The child's point of view. *Journal of Social Service Research, 1*(1), 77-92.

Goldstein, A. P., Sprafkin, R. P., Gershaw, N. J., & Klein, P. (1980). *Skillstreaming the adolescent.* Champaign, IL: Research Press.

Gould, L. (1969). Conformity and marginality: Two faces of alienation. *Journal of Social Issues, 25*(2), 39-63.

Graham, J. W., Flay, B. R., Johnson, C. A., Hansen, W. B., Grossman, L., & Sobel, J. L. (1984). Reliability of self-report measures of drug use in prevention research: Evaluation of the Project Smart Questionnaire vs. Test-Retest Reliability Matrix. *Journal of Drug Education, 14*(2).

Gurney, B. G. (1977). *Relationship enhancement.* San Francisco: Jossey-Bass.

Hops, H., Willis, T., Patterson, G. R., & Weiss, R. L. (1972). *Marital interaction coding system (MICS).* University of Oregon and Oregon Research Institute (NAPS Document 02077), Eugene, OR.

Horan, J. J., & Williams, J. M. (1975). The tentative drug use scale: A quick and relatively problem free outcome measure for drug abuse prevention projects. *Journal of Drug Education, 5*(4), 381-384.

Hudson, W. W. (1982). *The clinical measurement package: A field manual.* Chicago: Dorsey Press.

Hudson, W. W., Acklin, J. D., & Bartosh, J. C. (1980). Assessing discord in family relationships. *Social Work Research and Abstracts, 16*(3), 21-29.

Hudson, W. W., Wung, B., & Borges, M. (1980). Parent-child relationship disorders: The parent's point of view. *Journal of Social Service Research, 3*(3), 283-294.

Jesness, C. F. (1969). *The Jesness Inventory manual.* Palo Alto, CA: Consulting Psychologist Press.

Kaplan, R. M., Konecni, V. J., & Novaco, R. W. (Eds.). (1984). *Aggression in children and youth* (No. 17 in the NATO Advanced Science Institute Series, "Behavioural and Social Sciences."). The Hague, The Netherlands: Martinus Nijhoff.

Kirby, D. (1984). *Sexual education: An evaluation of programs and their effects.* CA: Network Publications.

Lange, A. J., & Jakubowski, P. (1976). *Responsible assertive behavior.* Champaign, IL: Research Press.

Lettieri, D. J. (1981). Recommendations from a science administration perspective. In *Assessing marijuana consequences: Selected questionnaire items* (pp. 111-128). Washington, DC: U. S. Department of Health and Human Services, National Institute on Drug Abuse.

Lewinsohn, P. M., Antonuccio, D. O., Steinmetz, J. L., & Teri, L. (1984). *The coping with depression course.* Eugene, OR: Castalia Publishing.

McMahon, R. J., Forehand, R. L., & Griest, D. L. (1981). Effects of knowledge of social learning principles on enhancing treatment outcome and generalization in a parent training program. *Journal of Consulting and Clinical Psychology, 49,* 526-532.

Meyer, R. G., & Smith, S. S. (1977). A crisis in group therapy. *American Psychologist, 32,* 638-643.

Novaco, R. W. (1975). *Anger control: The development and evaluation of an experimental treatment.* Lexington, MA: Lexington Books, D. C. Heath & Co.

O'Dell, S. L., Tarler-Benlolo, L., & Flynn, J. M. (1977). *An instrument to measure knowledge of behavioral principles as applied to children.* Unpublished manuscript, Nova University.

Olson, D. H., McCubbin, H. I., Barnes, H., Larsen, A., Muxen, M., & Wilson, M. (1982). *Family inventories: Inventories used in a national survey of families across the family life cycle.* St. Paul: University of Minnesota, Family Social Science.

Platt, J. J., & Spivack, G. (1975). *The Means-Ends Problem Solving Procedure manual.* Philadelphia: Hahnemann University, Department of Mental Health Services.

Platt, J. J., Spivack, G., Altman, N., & Altman, D. (1974). Adolescent problem-solving thinking. *Journal of Consulting and Clinical Psychology, 42,* 787-793.

Prinz, R. J., Foster, S., Kent, R. N., & O'Leary, K. D. (1979). Multivariate assessment of conflict in distressed and nondistressed mother-adolescent dyads. *Journal of Applied Behavior Analysis, 12,* 691-700.

Quay, H. C., & Peterson, D. R. (1983). *Interim manual for the revised behavior problem checklist.* Unpublished manual.

Reid, W. J. (1978). *The task-centered system.* New York: Columbia University Press.

Reynolds, W. M. (1985, March). *Development and validation of a scale to measure depression in adolescents.* Paper presented at the annual meeting of the Society for Personality Assessment, Berkeley, CA.

Reynolds, W. M. (1986). *Assessment of depression in adolescents: Manual for the Reynolds Adolescent Depression Scale.* Odessa, FL: Psychological Assessment Resources.

Robin, A. L., & Foster, S. L. (1984). Problem-solving communication training: A behavioral family systems approach to parent-adolescent conflict. In P. Karoly & J. Steffen (Eds.), *Adolescent behavior disorders: Foundations and contemporary concerns.* Lexington, MA: Lexington Books.

Robin, A. L., & Weiss, J. G. (1980). Criterion-related validity of behavioral and self-report measures of problem-solving communication skills in distressed and non-distressed parent-adolescent dyads. *Behavioral Assessment, 2,* 339-352.

Rose, S. D. (1977). *Group therapy: A behavioral approach.* Englewood Cliffs, NJ: Prentice-Hall.

Ross, H., & Glaser, E. (1973). Making it out of the ghetto. *Professional Psychology, 4*(3), 347-356.

Rusch, F. R., (1986). Identifying and teaching social behaviors. In F. Rusch (Ed.), *Competitive employment issues and strategies* (pp.273-282). Baltimore: Paul H. Brookes.

Schinke, S. P., & Gilchrist, L. D. (1984). *Life skills counseling with adolescents.* Baltimore: University Park Press.

Siegel, J. M., Platt, J. J., & Peizer, S. B. (1976). Emotional and social real-life problem solving thinking in adolescent and adult psychiatric patients. *Journal of Clinical Psychology, 32*(2), 230-232.

Smith, K. A., & Forehand, R. L. (in press). Parent-adolescent conflict: Comparison and prediction of the perceptions of mothers, fathers, and daughters in a nonclinic sample. *Journal of Early Adolescence.*

Spence, S. H., & Marzillier, J. S. (1981). Social skills training with adolescent male offenders: II. Short-term, long-term and generalized effects. *Behaviour Research and Therapy, 19*, 349-368.

Spielberger, C. D. (1983). *State-Trait Anxiety Inventory.* Palo Alto, CA: Consulting Psychologists Press.

Spivack, G., & Shure, M. B. (1974). *Social adjustment of young children.* San Francisco: Jossey-Bass.

Wodarski, J. S. (1981). *Role of research in clinical practice.* Austin, TX: PRO-ED.

Wodarski, J. S., & Bagarozzi, D. A. (1979). *Behavioral social work.* New York: Human Sciences Press.

Wodarski, L. A., Adelson, C. L., Tidball, M. T., & Wodarski, J. S. (1980). Teaching nutrition by teams-games-tournaments. *Journal of Nutrition Education, 12*(2), 61-65.

Zung, W. W. K. (1974). *The measurement of depression.* Summit, NJ: CIBA Pharmaceutical Company.

Chapter 4

TEENAGE PREGNANCY: THE SOCIAL DILEMMA OF THE EIGHTIES IMPLICATIONS FOR SOCIAL WORK PRACTICE

Lettie L. Lockhart and John S. Wodarski

INTRODUCTION

ONE OF THE critical social problems facing our society is the marked increase in the number of adolescents who have become parents but are insufficiently mature, and are unable or unwilling to provide adequate care, protection, and nurturing that a child needs (Crawford & Furstenberg, 1985). A recent report by the Guttmacher Institute (1985) revealed that 40 percent of today's 14-year-old girls can expect to become pregnant by the time they are 20 years old. Each year roughly 600,000 babies are born to the one million teenage girls who become pregnant (Guttmacher Institute, 1985), approximately 378,500 are aborted and the remainder are recorded as stillbirths or miscarriages (Dryfoos, 1982a, 1982b; National Center for Health Statistics, 1978). Furthermore, more than half of these adolescent mothers will have a repeat pregnancy within two years after the birth of their first child (while they are still school age) which heightens their probability for societal dependency (Howard, 1978; Trussell & Menken, 1978).

These statistics speak plainly to the magnitude of the problem. Adolescents who become pregnant are ensuring for themselves and their babies a bleak future. A future marked by truncated education, inadequate vocational training, poor work skills, economic dependency and poverty, large single-parent households and social isolation (Barth & Schinke, 1983). As Campbell (1968) commented earlier in our societal concern over this problem, 90 percent of an adolescent's life script is written when she becomes a mother, and the story is often an unhappy one.

Adolescent pregnancy is increasingly commonplace today and poses many difficulties for both the individuals involved and society as a whole. For programs to successfully address this problem, factors related to unintended pregnancies and consequences of teenagers' pregnancies must be identified and understood. Thus, this chapter is a review of current literature on these factors and consequences. Additionally, an examination of relevant prevention strategies will be examined in order to provide a rationale for the need for a more comprehensive practice model to prevent teenage pregnancies which is elaborated in this chapter.

FACTORS RELATED TO TEENAGE PREGNANCIES

Physiological Changes and Changes in Incidence Rates

A decrease in the average age at which the menstrual cycle begins and increasing sexual activity among youths have resulted in an alarmingly high incidence of teenage pregnancy (Chilman, 1979; Flick, 1986; Schinke, 1978). Sexual activity most often begins before the sixteenth year. Many youths sexually debut before they are 13 (Baldwin, 1980). Forty percent more black than white teenagers have been sexually active (Zelnik & Kantner, 1980), but fewer blacks than whites have many partners and fewer blacks have intercourse very frequently (Zelnik & Kantner, 1977). Sexual activity is increasing most rapidly among white adolescents (Zelnik & Kantner, 1980).

Contraceptive Use

Contraceptive use has not kept pace with adolescents' coital activity. Many sexually active youths wait a year or more before requesting birth control information and/or services (De Amicis, Klorman, Hess, & McAnarney, 1981). Despite widespread availability of over-the-counter contraceptives such as condoms, foams, and sponges, only one out of three adolescents aged 15 to 19 uses contraceptives each time he or she has intercourse. Contraceptive use also seems to decrease with age (Zelnik & Kantner, 1980). Developmentally, adolescents are at a cognitive stage in their lives that may make contraceptive use less likely, i.e. guilt is associated with the predeterminance of birth control. To avoid pregnancy, adolescents must have the cognitive ability to think abstractly — to connect present with future consequences — and must be able to logically consider possible solutions and to recognize the risks involved in unprotected sexual experiences (Doctors, 1985; Urburg, 1982). Adolescents (especially the younger ones) have not achieved this level of cognitive ability (Cobliner, 1974).

Additional significant reasons for failure of adolescents to use birth control methods (especially the most effective ones) are disquieting (De Amicis et al., 1981; Nadelson, Hatman, & Gellon, 1980; Zelnik & Kantner, 1979). Many adolescents do not really believe contraception methods work as reflected by the figures that one-third of the pregnant teens in the Furstenberg et al. (1968) study agreed with the statements that: "Birth control doesn't work, even if you're careful" and "Even if I could, I don't think I would want to use birth control every time I had intercourse" (p. 39). Nadelson and his colleagues (1980) as well as Zelnik and Kantner (1979) reported that one-third to one-half of the adolescents they studied believed that they or their partners could not get pregnant due to their age, the time of the month of intercourse, and their limited number of sexual contacts. Adolescent pregnancy may be affected by attitudes, beliefs, and/or maturation. Pregnancy may have certain positive connotations and denotations for adolescents. That is, it may falsely confirm the womanhood (and fertility) for females and the virility (or manhood) of the males (Stiffman & Morse, 1986).

Increased use of birth control is found in adolescents who have higher levels of communication between partners (Anderson, McPherson, Beeching, Weinberg, & Vessey, 1978; Cvetkovich & Grote, 1980), and higher levels of parent-child communication about sexual activities and birth control (Fox & Inazu, 1980; Herald & Samson, 1980). Adolescents who are successful users of contraception methods are more likely to have accurate information about sex and contraception, higher academic achievement and exhibit a stronger sense of individual and internal locus of control (Mindick & Oskamp, 1982).

Family Communication

Most Americans believe that it is desirable for parents to discuss sexual issues and contraception with their children, but such communication occurs so infrequently. Thus, families are logical places for investigating factors that lead adolescents toward and away from the risk of early pregnancies (Schinke, 1984). For example, Bloch (1974) reported one out of every five mothers of seventh grade girls who participated in his study had not explained menstruation to their daughters, one-half of them had never alluded to the male's role in reproduction, and two-thirds of these mothers had never discussed birth control. Fox (1980) studied communication about sexual behaviors and concerns between parent and child and found that greater frequency of mother-daughter communication about sexual questions was associated with more responsible patterns of the daughter's sexual behavior (Cicirelli, 1980). He further contended that frequent discussions made possible a kind of "anticipatory rehearsal" which allowed the daughter to accept her sexuality and desensitize the topics of sex and birth control, to the extent that discussions about responsible sexual behavior could also occur between daughter and partner.

These data support assertions that children get little sex education at home. Many families head off the discussion of sexual matters through a "conspiracy of silence"—they may even suspect the worst is happening, but they'd rather hope for the best and keep silent (Lindemann, 1974; Pocs, Godow, Tolone, & Walsh, 1977, p. 56). Researchers of mother-daughter communication have suggested that a potential for positive familial influence on this subject matter has largely gone untapped (Cicirelli, 1980; Fox & Inazu, 1980; Olson & Worsbey, 1984; Sheehy, 1974). Cicirelli (1980) indicated that mother-daughter relations make a difference in strongly influencing adolescents' sexual behaviors. He contends that girls are more strongly influenced by parents than boys, and there is evidence to suggest that mothers are (can be) the major force in girls' lives. In support of Cicirelli's assertions, Fox and Inazu (1980) reported that the strongest predictor of sexual experience was the daughter's report of her relationship with her mother; the more favorable the relationship, the less likely was the daughter to engage in premarital sex (p. 28).

Peer Influence

Peer groups greatly influence sexual behavior which is not always helpful in shaping teenagers' sexual attitudes and behavior (Cvetkovich & Grote, 1980; Rosenberg, 1980; Zelnik & Shah, 1983). Rosenberg (1980) reported that teenagers are most likely to discuss sex and birth control with friends, with whom they may well have exchanged inaccurate information. Rosenberg further reported that the knowledge teenagers had on topics such as masturbation, ejaculation, petting, intercourse, prostitution, homosexuality and contraceptives generally came from their peers. When it came to birth control information received from friends, only one in five teenagers in Rosenberg's study was accurately knowledgeable (Schinke, 1984). A high involvement with peers and strong resemblance of peer values and views as opposed to parents often overrides the effects of parental involvement for adolescent males and is also associated with early sexual behavior for both gender groups (Miller & Simon, 1974; Zelnik & Shah, 1983). Studies have also indicated that teenagers' perceptions of frequent coital activities by peers or awareness of peers who use birth control is strongly associated with greater sexual activity (Cvetkovich & Grote, 1980; Hansson, O'Conner, Jones, & Blocker, 1981; Jorgenson, King, & Torrey, 1980). Peer influences were also reported by female adolescents who had sex because they felt unable to say no, wanted to please their partners, or saw intercourse as expected at the end of a date, and were reported by teenage males who said they initiated coitus to prove their love (Cvetkovich & Grote, 1980; Field, 1981; Rogel & Zuehlke, 1982).

Adolescents at Risk

Adolescents who engage in sexual activities are also those who are most likely to be impulsive risk takers and to participate in "deviant behavior such as alcohol or drug use or other delinquent behavior" (Jessor & Jessor, 1985). They have lower grades in school, lower expectations of achievements, lower acceptance of parental controls and are more likely to see their parents and friends as being in conflict. Many adolescent mothers have a low sense of self-esteem and levels of competence, poor individual and internal locus of control, and are more inclined to be passive and hold traditional stereotypical views of male-female gender roles (Cvetkovich & Grote, 1980; Cvetkovich, Grote, Lieberman, & Miller, 1978; Jessor & Jessor, 1975, 1985; Miller & Simon, 1974). Regular church attendance and/or association with an established religion has also been negatively associated with sexual activities of adolescents (Chilman, 1980; Jessor & Jessor, 1975, 1985; Miller & Simon, 1974).

CONSEQUENCES OF ADOLESCENT PREGNANCY

Health

Teenage pregnancies are associated with substantially increased health risks for both the mother and child. Adolescent pregnancies that result in childbirth often result in severe, adverse consequences such as high incidences of pregnancy and childbirth complications, and high incidences of low birth weight babies which are often associated with developmental and mental disabilities and high infant mortality and morbidity rates (Bolton, 1980; Levering, 1983; Rutter, 1980). Low birth weight and infant death are twice as likely for adolescent mothers than those beyond their teen years. These babies are also two to three times more likely to die in their first year as compared to babies born to older women (Hunt, 1976). Pregnancy-related health risks faced by adolescent girls may be attributed to biological immaturity, nutritionally insufficient diets and poor prenatal care (Klerman & Jekel, 1973; Septo, Keith, & Keith, 1975; Ventura & Hendershort, 1984).

Interpersonal

Children of adolescent mothers are at greater risk of abuse and neglect. Studies have indicated a significant negative correlation between the age of the mother and the potential for abuse and gross neglect of the child (Helfer & Kempe, 1972). Additionally, children of teenage mothers are more likely to become teenage mothers themselves and continuing this cycle of recurring abuse and early childbearing (American Humane Association, 1978; Bolton, Laner, & Kane, 1980; Herrenkohl & Herrenkohl, 1979). Social and psychological studies further indicate that behavior disorders, school problems, and low intellectual functioning are more probable for adolescents' offspring than children of non-adolescent mothers. Many of the social and psychological problems are largely attributable to the social and economic insecurities of these teenage mothers (Belmont, Stein, & Zybert, 1978; Finkelstein, Finkelstein, Christie, Roden, & Shelton, 1982; Gunter & La Barba, 1980).

Moreover, psychologically, the role change from teenager to mother can produce negative emotional experiences. The unwed pregnant teenager who decides to have and keep her baby is often unprepared for the ensuing isolation and extremely demanding role of motherhood (Chilman, 1980; Gilchrist & Schinke, 1983a, 1983b; Quay, 1981). Adolescent years are known for the "emotional turbulence." Teenagers are still developing the coping skills and maturity needed for a psychologically healthy life—which have not fully developed—but are necessary for positive parenting (Levering, 1983; Little & Kendall, 1979; Smith, Weinman, & Mumford, 1982). At its worst, emotional stresses and depression experienced by many adolescent mothers lead to frustration and anger which could ultimately be vented through violence either to themselves or their children. Gabrielson and his colleagues (1970) reported a higher incidence of suicide among pregnant adolescents.

Employment Preparation

Adolescent pregnancy, for those girls who become parents and keep their children, interrupts and/or terminates education, which results in reduced earning power and dependence on public assistance and the social welfare system (Furstenberg, 1980; Levering, 1983; Moore & Caldwell, 1977; Trussell & Menken, 1978). Data from the Wodarski, Parham, Lindsey and Blackburn (1986) study entitled "Toward a Poverty Agenda" indicates that this may be one of the most significant factors involved in welfare dependency. Teenage parents encounter additional stresses of ill-considered marriages and an increased likelihood of marital problems and high divorce rates (Lorenzi, Klerman, & Jekel, 1977).

Early parenthood has a disruptive effect on education which in turn affects subsequent job opportunities and income levels when these parents keep their children. The new responsibilities as a parent also interfere with the young mother's ability to locate employment (Kamerman, 1985). The odds for an adolescent mother achieving a successful and rewarding life are significantly lower than for those women who postpone childbearing until they are at least 20 years old. The very young woman often falls into a "syndrome of failure" which is hard to stop. Her combined lack of education, skills and work experience makes a poor resume for future employment and often leads to economic dependency (Burden & Klerman, 1984; Dillard & Pol, 1982, p. 257).

Furthermore, adolescent mothers tend to have repeat pregnancies which only serve to perpetuate this "syndrome of failure" (Schinke, 1984). The odds of falling into this syndrome are great, especially since 80 percent or more of adolescent mothers, age 17 or younger, do not finish high school. What are her options? Welfare is one possibility and marriage is another. Sixty percent of women in single-headed households receive AFDC and had their first child while in their teens (Kamerman, 1985). Adolescent mothers fall below federal poverty lines—twice the rate of women who initiate childbearing after their teen years (Barker, Loughlin, & Rudolph, 1979). Reducing the number of subsequent pregnancies of young mothers is one of the major factors in reducing long-term dependency (Bane & Ellwood, 1983, p. vii).

Some of the immediate economic problems are solved when teenage mothers have a strong social support system, e.g. family and parents. Many of these teen mothers stay with their parents or relatives, at least for a period of time (Scheirer, 1983; U. S. Bureau of the Census, 1983). Thus, because poverty rates for teenage mothers who head their household is very high, most teenage mothers live as subfamilies in the household of a relative, usually a parent (Kamerman, 1985). Because many teenage mothers come from families who are economically disadvantaged themselves, this too causes additional stress and strain that could cause family tension or dissolution (Howard, 1978; Kamerman, 1985).

APPROACHES TO PREVENTION

Past Approaches to Prevention

Despite extensive documentation of early childbearing consequences, efforts to prevent or ameliorate teenage pregnancy have been ineffective. One reason for this failure appears to be the lack of a complete conceptual framework of understanding and preventing this growing social problem. An extensive literature review reveals that recent approaches to understand and prevent teenage pregnancy can be characterized as either a reductionistic model stressing a single underlying explanation, or a developmental model emphasizing a normal adolescent maturational process (Schinke & Gilchrist, 1977). The reductionistic approach explains teenage pregnancy as resulting from one problem condition/factor which leads to a single, straightforward assumption: given easy low-cost access to sex and contraceptive education and services, adolescents will be informed, responsible and self-regulating in avoiding unplanned pregnancies. Prevention as emphasized in traditional sex education attempts to change attitudes by exposing adolescents to unattractive consequences of their behaviors. This so-called "scare tactic" approach has not been effective in preventing teenage pregnancies (Dryfoos, 1983; Gilchrist, Schinke, & Blythe, 1979).

Search for a pathology that underlies teenage sexual activities has directed many efforts and has guided much of the reductionistic prevention programs. Researchers have looked for personality correlates of adolescents' vulnerability to intercourse (Goldfarb, Mumford, Schum, Smith, Flower, & Schum, 1977), pregnancy risk (Rosen & Ager, 1981), and decision making about childbearing (Perlman, Klerman, & Kinard, 1981). Research has uncovered little reason to suspect that adolescents' sexual behavior is pathological (Gilchrist, 1981; Gilchrist & Schinke, 1983a, 1983b; Litt, Cuskey, & Rudd, 1980; Olson, 1980; Schinke, 1979). Nevertheless, a host of social service programs for teenagers have been based on the pathological orientation. Thus, pathologically oriented sex education programs have had little or no effect on adolescents' sexual behavior (Kirby, 1980; Mindick & Oskamp, 1979; Reid, 1982; Zelnik & Kim, 1982).

The developmentalists have strongly stressed the complexity of interactional multiple factors that influence adolescents' behavior. They suggest that situational, social, interpersonal and maturational factors may interact to lead adolescents into premarital sexual activities, and can be factors that prevent adolescents from effectively applying their contraceptive knowledge and understanding (Cvetkovich & Grote, 1980; Sandberg & Jacobs, 1971). Cvetkovich and Grote (1980) further suggest that female adolescents may be placed at pregnancy risk "not by any form of pathology, moral or otherwise, but, by a unique convergence of factors which are 'normal' to the lives of many" (p. 2). Adolescence is a period of growth, which demands mastery of critical developmental tasks, two of which are learning sexual functioning (Wagner, 1970) and the relational nature of sexual activities (McAlister, Perry, & Maccoby, 1979). McAlister and his colleagues (1979) suggest that if prevention efforts are to be effective, their developers must consider factors which include the interpersonal aspects of risk taking, the social significance of many problem behaviors, and the role of peer pressure. In the Cvetkovich and Grote study (1980), females reported they became sexually active because they could not say no, because they wanted to please and satisfy their boyfriends, or because it seemed as though sexual activity was expected of them.

One major perspective of this approach suggests that adolescents acquire cognitive and behavioral skills to cope with the new opportunities and expectations accompanying physical and social maturity, if they are to avoid behaviors detrimental to themselves and others. Additionally, this perspective suggests that adolescents need skills to transform knowledge or abstract information into personal decisions and personal decisions into overt behavior (Schinke, Gilchrist & Blythe, 1980; Schinke, Gilchrist, & Small, 1979).

A second perspective used under the developmentalistic approach is the values clarification perspective (Chesler, 1980). Chesler (1980) suggested, "In addition to needing accurate, unbiased information about contraceptive technology, teenagers need help in clarifying their values so that their social behaviors are congruent with their moral codes" (p. 18). Although the data are not in, value-focused programs, aimed at values clarification, may have the potential of lowering teenage pregnancy and of transferring values to other developmental tasks teenagers are confronted with during this stage (Toohey & Valenzuela, 1982). Earlier research, however, on values clarification programs has indicated that this perspective has not helped teenagers improve their self-esteem, changed their interpersonal relationships, or altered their sexual values and/or behavior (Lockwood, 1978).

Current Prevention Strategies

Prevention programs may be classified into three general groups: sex education and information, contraceptive services, and the broadening of life options such as general education and employment during pregnancy and after childbirth (Dryfoos, 1983). Sex education is considered the primary prevention strategy of teenage pregnancy.

Sex education is one prevention strategy of teenage pregnancy that offers two great advantages: it can reach all young people before they become sexually active, and information can be provided to them at relatively low cost through the school, churches and other delivery systems. In the past, sex education attempted to help adolescents understand the physical changes accompanying puberty, the biology of reproduction and the responsibilities of family life. Today, however, most Americans believe sex education should address the complex problems of human sexuality that teenagers face. But a few people still believe that sex education, particularly when it covers methods of contraception, actually increases teenagers' sexuality, causes an upswing in unintended pregnancies, and undermines the family unit (Kenney & Orr, 1984). Consequently, sex education remains controversial, despite the enormous diversity of nationwide program offerings. Parents and teenagers believe, however, that sex education plays an important role in the prevention of unwanted teenage pregnancies (Bachman, Johnston, & O'Malley, 1980; Gallup Opinion Index, 1978).

If adolescents are to adopt the idea of pregnancy prevention, then sex education strategies must be an integral part of a youth's development and should begin before the onset of puberty (McAnarney & Schreider, 1984). In practice, most sex education curricula and programs have occurred too late in the developmental cycle, focusing on high school and college students (Blythe, Gilchrist, & Schinke, 1981; Gilchrist & Schinke, 1983a, 1983b; Gilchrist, Schinke, & Blythe, 1979; Schinke, 1982; Schinke, Blythe, Gilchrist, & Burt, 1981).

Sex education rarely involves parents as primary sex educators of their children (McAnarney & Schreider, 1984). Research has revealed that fewer than 1 in 5 parents tell their teenage children about intercourse, discuss birth controls or provide them with sex education literature (Schinke & Gilchrist, 1984). McAnarney and her associates (1984) suggest several reasons for this: (1) parents may not have adequate information to share; (2) parents may not know how to educate their child about sexuality; (3) parents may be uncomfortable with the subject; and (4) adolescents may be uncomfortable when parents assume the role of sex educator, especially if no discussion of the subject has occurred before puberty. Parents need to be prepared for their role as sex educators before their children reach teenage years.

Very few sex education programs have been systematically evaluated (Kirby, 1985). Virtually no attempts have been made to conduct follow-up studies to ascertain the long-term effects of sex education on students' knowledge, attitudes, and behavior. Evaluative studies of sex education have concluded that there was no evidence to support the belief that sex education will increase or decrease sexual activities of teenagers (Kirby, Alter, & Scales, 1979), or to support the claim that the decision to engage in sexual activities is influenced by sex education in school. However, females who are sexually active and had sex education that covered contraceptive methods appeared somewhat more likely to use contraceptives the first time they engaged in sexual intercourse and experience fewer pregnancies than sexually active females who did not have formal sex education (Zelnik & Kim, 1982). A needed element of evaluative research of sex education programs is the study of the long-term retention of knowledge.

New Directions: The Comprehensive Parent, Peers and School Prevention Model

Acknowledgment of a problem is the first step toward its resolution. Substantial research has been devoted to teenage pregnancy. Individuals who are associated with youths can demonstrate their concern to combat the problem of teenage pregnancy through developing prevention programs aimed at three groups: adolescents, parents, and school teachers and counselors. For effective pregnancy prevention training, information input and behavior change output must be considered. More important, training must address influential intervening variables—cognitive and moral processes mediating the understanding and use of information in decision making. Thus, a comprehensive education program that gives teenagers, parents, and school teachers/counselors accurate sex education through a curriculum that is attractive, social skills training in terms of assertiveness and problem solving, and practice applying this information in at-risk situations is needed.

Timing and Educational Content

Research has indicated that if adolescents are to adopt the idea of pregnancy prevention, then sex education must be an integral part of youths' personal development and begin before or during puberty (McAnarney & Schreider, 1984; Thornburg, 1981). The introduction of sex education prevention programs at the middle school level would be appropriate. This follows the suggestion by Jorgensen and Alexander (1983) that sex education programs must begin to span preadolescence, early adolescence and adolescence, in order to circumvent our traditional practices of providing "too little, too late" to have an impact on adolescent pregnancy rates. Programs could be incorporated into a health education course, group discussions at local youth groups associated with churches as well as other formal and informal community organizations (Doty & King, 1985).

Although it is often said that sex education programs should be value-free, Scales (1983) and McAnarney and Schreider (1984) have pointed out that sex education is not value-free. Each program and community, including parents, will stress their own beliefs which are embodied in the program's goals (Scales, 1983). Therefore, the program is grounded in a set of values. Students need not agree initially with these values, but they should be clearly stated so that they can make decisions against a known standard. The following values will be incorporated into the sex education program:

1. Being a teen parent is not a good idea, it brings with it social, emotional, educational, financial and medical consequences.
2. No one should be pressured into a sexual act against his/her will or principles.
3. Postponement of sexual intercourse should be strongly encouraged until they have at least completed high school.

4. The double standards for males and females, which still exists in our society, is not to be condoned.
5. Having unprotected intercourse is like skydiving without a parachute — it is politically, socially, emotionally and financially suicidal.

Peers

Prevention programs should assist adolescents to identify and examine peer pressure and explore ways to make individual, deliberate decisions, especially since peers have significant impact on each other's behaviors. Thus, we posit that sex education should be offered through a peer group experience. Peer learning structures should create a learning situation in which the performance of each group member furthers the attainment of overall group goals. This increases individual members' support for group performance, strengthens performance under a variety of similar circumstances, and further enhances the attainment of group-goals. Group reward structures capitalize on peer influence and peer reinforcement. These are considered to be some of the most potent variables in the acquisition, alteration, and maintenance of prosocial norms among youths (Buckholdt & Wodarski, 1978). Peer programs that foster the adolescent's sense of self-worth, awareness of one's own feelings, and assertiveness will help adolescents learn to act in their own interest, with a stronger sense of control over their own lives. Moreover, because of the important role of adolescent males, a prevention program must be aimed at males as well as females. Adolescent males are presently less aware of the risks of pregnancy, less informed about contraceptives, less supportive of the use of contraceptives than females and they have the most to learn from a sex education program (Freeman, 1978).

Parent Component

Parents greatly influence their children's behavior. Next to peers, parental involvement and communication should be strengthened to help adolescents become more responsible. In a 1979 survey by Yankelovich, Skelly and White, Inc. (1979), 84 percent of the parents of teenagers said it was up to them to teach their children about sex-related topics even though they supported sex education in public schools. Although parents want to be involved in educating their children about sexually related topics, they find it very difficult (Fox, 1980; Fox & Inazu, 1980). Parents need the skills to establish open communication with their children regarding sexual issues. The main thrust of the program with parents should be on heightening communication skills between parents and children, since lack of communication consistently has been shown to have an effect on teenage sexual activities (Cvetkovich & Grote, 1980; Fox & Inazu, 1980; McAnarney & Schreider, 1984). Focusing on increasing parents' skills in communicating, especially in the areas of value clarification or moral consciousness, the relational aspect of sexuality as well as other sexually related topics should be a major part of the program for the parental group of the prevention model. Parental involvement in prevention programs is needed to help parents, who are often less informed than their teenagers (Dryfoos, 1982a, 1982b), become more informed and comfortable with discussing sexual issues with their children. Parental involvement is a necessary element of any successful prevention model so that accurate and open communication as well as the learning process can be supported at home. Fathers should be present with their sons and mothers with their daughters.

SUMMARY

In order to alleviate the dilemma of teenagers having children, it is evident that the following requisites are necessary.

(1) Timing of sex education is critical and should occur in the middle school years.

(2) Attractive curriculums taught by qualified teachers are necessary.

(3) The incorporation of the peer group experience as a learning vehicle is also necessary, since peer norms influence sexual behavior.

(4) An essential aspect of sex education should involve the opportunity to practice appropriate behaviors for high-risk situations.

(5) A final component to the comprehensive model should be the involvement of parents in the education of their children.

One of the reasons why sex education has failed our youngsters is that we have not employed enough foci for making it meaningful to them. The solution to the problem of pregnancy among teens requires an all out effort by those societal forces capable of effecting change. Families, schools, peers, communities, businesses and the media all possess powers to erradicate this social problem. The campaign cannot be waged from only one front; however, combined, cooperative efforts are essential. The responsibility must be shared for both previous condoning of actions that have perpetuated the problem and for working toward mutual goals and solutions.

It is time for social work to deal preventively with the epidemic of teenage pregnancy. For years social workers have been aware of the rapidly increasing rate of teenage pregnancy. They know through their practice experiences the negative social, emotional and financial consequences many of these early pregnancies bring to families (Gordon & Dickman, 1980). For years social workers have responded to this problem by developing programs for girls who are parents or pregnant, but few social work programs serve both boys and girls with a focus on preventing pregnancy. Too often, teenagers are offered information and counseling about sexual issues only after a problem has developed (Doty & King, 1985).

Social workers have the necessary skills and sensitivity to carry out comprehensive sex education and counseling programs that involve the schools and parents in a partnership in sex education. Social work is in a unique position to initiate this comprehensive school/parent partnership in sex education, since social workers have traditionally worked with families and school systems in coordinating multifaceted services. Social workers are extremely knowledgeable and skillful in the areas of interpersonal relationships and decision making as well as issues of human sexuality. The model offered in this chapter offers the profession the ability to continue to serve as the nation's social conscience regarding this major societal problem.

This chapter reviewed the scope of teenage pregnancy. Next, a discussion of the factors related to teenage pregnancy occurred in terms of physiological changes and changes in incidence rates, contraceptive use, family communication, peer influence and adolescents at risk. The consequences of adolescent pregnancy were elaborated in terms of health, interpersonal skills and employment preparation. Past approaches to prevention were discussed and new approaches were reviewed. The chapter concluded with a presentation of a comprehensive prevention model involving parents, peers and schools.

REFERENCES

American Humane Association. (1978). *National analysis of official child neglect and abuse reporting: An executive summary.* Englewood, CO: American Humane Association.

Anderson, P., McPherson, K., Beeching, N., Weinberg, J., & Vessey, M. (1978). Sexual behavior and contraceptive practice of undergraduates at Oxford University. *Journal of Biosocial Science, 10*(3), 277-286.

Bachman, J. G., Johnston, L. D., & O'Malley, P. M. (1980). *Monitoring the future: Questionnaire responses from the nation's high school seniors, 1978.* Ann Arbor: University of Michigan Institute for Social Research, Survey Research Center.

Baldwin, W. H. (1980). Adolescent pregnancy and childbearing: Growing concerns for Americans. *Population Bulletin, 31*(2), 1-37.

Bane, M. J., & Ellwood, D. T. (1983). *The dynamics of dependence: The routes to self-sufficiency* (prepared for the Office of Income Security Policy, U. S. Department of Health and Human Services). Washington, DC: U. S. Government Printing Office.

Barker, S. R., Loughlin, J., & Rudolph, C. S. (1979). The long-term effects of adolescent childbearing: A retrospective analysis. *Journal of Social Service Research, 2*(4), 341-355.

Barth, R. P., & Schinke, S. P. (1983). Coping with daily strain among pregnant and parenting adolescents. *Journal of Social Service Research, 7*(2), 51-63.

Belmont, L., Stein, Z., & Zybert, P. (1978). Child spacing and birth order: Effect on intellectual ability in two-child families. *Science, 202*(4371), 995-996.

Bloch, D. (1974). Sex education practices of mothers. *Journal of Sex Education and Therapy, 7,* 7-12.

Blythe, B. J., Gilchrist, L. D., & Schinke, S. P. (1981). Pregnancy-prevention groups for adolescents. *Social Work, 26*(6), 503-504.

Bolton, F. G. (1980). *The pregnant adolescent: Problems of premature parenthood.* Beverly Hills, CA: SAGE Publications.

Bolton, F. G., Laner, R. H., & Kane, S. P. (1980). Child maltreatment risk among adolescent mothers: A study of reported cases. *American Journal of Orthopsychiatry, 50*(3), 489-504.

Buckholdt, D., & Wodarski, J. S. (1978). The effects of different reinforcement systems on cooperative behavior exhibited by children in classroom contexts. *Journal of Research and Development in Education, 12*(1), 50-68.

Burden, D. S., & Klerman, L. V. (1984). Teenage parenthood: Factors that lessen economic dependence. *Social Work, 29*(1), 11-16.

Campbell, A. (1968). The role of family in the reduction of poverty. *Journal of Marriage and the Family, 30*(2), 236-246.

Chesler, J. S. (1980). Twenty-seven strategies for teaching contraception to adolescents. *Journal of School Health, 50*(1), 18-21.

Chilman, C. S. (1979). *Adolescent sexuality in a changing American society: Social and psychological perspectives.* Washington, DC: U. S. Government Printing Office.

Chilman, C. S. (1980). Social and psychological research concerning adolescent childbearing: 1970-1980. *Journal of Marriage and the Family, 42*(4), 793-805.

Cicirelli, V. G. (1980). A comparison of college women's feelings toward their siblings and parents. *Journal of Marriage and the Family, 42*(1), 111-117.

Cobliner, W. G. (1974). Pregnancy in the single adolescent girl: The role of cognitive functions. *Journal of Youth and Adolescence, 3*(1), 17-29.

Crawford, A. G., & Furstenberg, F. F. (1985). Teenage sexuality, pregnancy, and childbearing. In Laird & Hartman (Eds.), *A handbook of child welfare: Context, knowledge and practice* (pp. 532-559). New York: The Free Press.

Cvetkovich, G., & Grote, B. (1980). Psychosocial development and the social problem of teenage illegitimacy. In C. Chilman (Ed.), *Adolescent pregnancy and childbearing: Findings from research* (pp. 15-41) [NIH Publication No. 81-2077]. Washington, DC: Department of Health and Human Services.

Cvetkovich, G., Grote, B., Lieberman, E., & Miller, W. (1978). Sex role development and teenage fertility-related behavior. *Adolescence, 13,* 231-236.

De Amicis, L. A., Klorman, R., Hess, D. N., & McAnarney, E. R. (1981). A comparison of unwed pregnant teenagers and nulligravid sexually active adolescents seeking contraception. *Adolescence, 16*(61), 11-20.

Dillard, K. D., & Pol, L. G. (1982). The individual economic cost of teenage childbearing. *Family Relations, 31*(2), 249-259.

Doctors, S. R. (1985). Premarital pregnancy and childbirth in adolescence: A psychological overview. In Z. De Fries, R. C. Friedman, & R. Corn (Eds.), *Sexuality: New perspectives* (pp. 45-70). Westport, CT: Greenwood Press.

Doty, M. B., & King, M. (1985). Pregnancy prevention: A private agency's program in public schools. *Social Work in Education, 7*(2), 90-99.

Dryfoos, J. G. (1982a). Contraceptive use, pregnancy intentions and pregnancy outcomes among U. S. women. *Family Planning Perspectives, 14*(2), 81-94.

Dryfoos, J. G. (1982b). The epidemiology of adolescent pregnancy: Incidence, outcomes, and interventions. In I. Stuart & C. Wells (Eds.), *Pregnancy in adolescence: Needs, problems, and management* (pp. 27-47). New York: Van Nostrand Reinhold Company.

Dryfoos, J. G. (1983). *Review of interventions in the field of prevention of adolescent pregnancy.* Preliminary report to the Rockefeller Foundation; Mimeograph.

Field, B. (1981). Socio-economic analysis of out of wedlock births among teenagers. In K. Scott, T. Field, & E. Robertson (Eds.), *Teenage parents and their offspring* (pp. 15-33). New York: Grune and Stratton.

Finkelstein, J. W., Finkelstein, J. A., Christie, M., Roden, M., & Shelton, C. (1982). Teenage pregnancy and parenthood: Outcome for mother and child. *Journal of Adolescent Health Care, 3*(1), 1-7.

Flick, L. H. (1986). Paths to adolescent parenthood: Implications for prevention. *Public Health Report, 101*(2), 132-147.

Fox, G. L. (1980). The mother-adolescent daughter relationship as a sexual socialization structure: A research review. *Family Relations, 29*(1), 21-80.

Fox, G. L., & Inazu, J. K. (1980). Patterns and outcomes of mother-daughter communication about sexuality. *Journal of Social Issues, 36*(1), 7-29.

Freeman, E. (1978). Abortion: Subjective attitudes and feelings. *Family Planning Perspectives, 10*(3), 150-155.

Furstenberg, F. F. (1980). Burdens and benefits: The impact of early childbearing on the family. *Journal of Social Issues, 36*(1), 64-87.

Furstenberg, F. F., Gordes, L., & Markowitz, M. (1968). Birth control knowledge and attitudes among unmarried pregnant adolescents: A preliminary report. *Journal of Marriage and the Family, 31*(1), 34-42.

Gabrielson, I. W., Klerman, L. V., Currie, J. B., Tyler, N. C., & Jekel, J. F. (1970). Suicide attempts in a population pregnant as teenagers. *American Journal of Public Health, 60*(12), 2289-2301.

Gallup opinion index, Report #156 (p. 28). (1978) Princeton, NJ: American Institute of Public Opinion.

Gilchrist, L. D. (1981). Group procedures for helping adolescents cope with sex. *Behavioral Group Therapy, 3*(1), 3-8.

Gilchrist, L. D., & Schinke, S. P. (1983a). Coping with contraception: Cognitive and behavioral methods with adolescents. *Cognitive Therapy and Research, 7*(5), 379-388.

Gilchrist, L. D., & Schinke, S. P. (1983b). Counseling with adolescents about their sexuality. In C. S. Chilman (Ed.), *Adolescent sexuality in a changing American society* (pp. 230-249). New York: Wiley.

Gilchrist, L. D., Schinke, S. P., & Blythe, B. J. (1979). Primary prevention services for children and youth. *Children and Youth Services Review, 1*(4), 379-391.

Goldfarb, J. L., Mumford, D. M., Schum, D. A., Smith, P. E., Flowers, C,, & Schum, C. (1977). An attempt to detect "pregnancy susceptibility" in indigent adolescent girls. *Journal of Youth and Adolescence, 6*(2), 127-143.

Gordon, S., & Dickman, I. R. (1980, May). *Schools and parents: Partners in sex education* (Public Affairs Pamphlet No. 581). New York: Public Affairs Committee.

Gunter, N. N., & La Barba, R. C. (1980). The consequences of adolescent childbearing on postnatal development. *International Journal of Behavioral Development, 3*(2), 191-214.

Guttmacher Institute. (1985, March 11). *Report on adolescent pregnancy.* New York: Guttmacher Institute.

Hansson, R., O'Conner, M., Jones, W., & Blocker, T. (1981). Maternal employment and adolescent sex behavior. *Journal of Youth and Adolescence, 10*(1), 55-60.

Helfer, R. E., & Kempe, C. H. (1972). The child's need for early recognition, immediate care and protection. In C. H. Kempe & R. E. Helfer (Eds.), *Helping the battered child and his family.* Philadelphia: J. B. Lippincott.

Herald, E. S., & Samson, L. M. (1980). Differences between women who begin pill use before and after first intercourse: Ontario, Canada. *Family Planning Perspectives, 12*(6), 304-305.

Herrenkohl, E. C., & Herrenkohl, R. C. (1979). A comparison of abused children and their nonabused siblings. *Journal of the American Academy of Child Psychiatry, 18*(2), 260-269.

Howard, M. (1978). Young parent families. In *Child welfare strategy in the coming years* (pp. 197-226) [DHEW Publication No. (OHDS) 78-30158]. Washington, DC: Office of Human Development Services, Administration for Children, Youth and Families.

Hunt, W. B. (1976). Adolescent fertility: Risk and consequences. *Population Reports,* 157-176.

Jessor, S. L., & Jessor, R. (1975). Transition from virginity to nonvirginity among youth: A social-psychological study over time. *Developmental Psychology, 11* 473-484.

Jessor, S. L., & Jessor, R. (1985). Structure of problem behavior in adolescence and young adulthood. *Journal of Consulting and Clinical Psychology, 53*(6), 890-904.

Jorgensen, S. R., & Alexander, S. J. (1983). Research on adolescent pregnancy risk: Implications for sex education programs. *Theory into Practice, 22*(2), 125-133.

Jorgensen, S. R., King, S. L., & Torrey, B. A. (1980). Dyadic and social network influences on adolescent exposure to pregnancy risk. *Journal of Marriage and the Family, 42*(1), 141-155.

Kamerman, S. B. (1985). Young, poor, a mother alone: Problems and possible solutions. In H. McAdoo & T. M. Parham (Eds.), *Services to young families: Program review and policy recommendations* (pp. 1-38). Washington, DC: American Public Welfare Association.

Kenney, A. M., & Orr, M. T. (1984). Sex education: An overview of current programs, policies, and research. *Phi Delta Kappan, 65*(7), 491-496.

Kirby, D. (1980). The effects of school sex education programs: A review of the literature. *Journal of School Health, 50*(10), 559-563.

Kirby, D. (1985). Sexuality education: A more realistic view of its effects. *Journal of School Health, 55*(10), 421-424.

Kirby, D., Alter, J., & Scales, P. (1979, July). *An analysis of U. S. sex education programs and evaluation methods* (DHEW Publication No. CD-2021-79-DKFR). Washington, DC: U. S. Department of Health, Education and Welfare.

Klerman, L., & Jekel, J. (1973). *School-age mothers: Problems, programs and policy.* Hamden, CT: Linnett.

Levering, C. S. (1983). Teenage pregnancy and parenthood. *Childhood Education, 59*(3), 182-185.

Lindemann, C. (1974). *Birth control and unmarried young women.* New York: Springer.

Litt, I. F., Cuskey, W. R., & Rudd, S. (1980). Identifying adolescents at risk for noncompliance with contraceptive therapy. *Journal of Pediatrics, 96*(4), 742-745.

Little, V. L., & Kendall, P. C. (1979). Cognitive-behavioral interventions with delinquents: Problem solving, role taking, and self-control. In P. Kendall & S. Hallon (Eds.), *Cognitive-behavioral interventions: Theory, research and procedures.* New York: Academic Press.

Lockwood, A. (1978). The effects of value clarification and moral development criteria. *Review of Educational Research, 48*(3), 325-364.

Lorenzi, M. E., Klerman, L. V., & Jekel, J. F. (1977). School-aged parents: How permanent a relationship? *Adolescence, 12*(45), 13-22.

McAlister, A. L., Perry, C., & Maccoby, N. (1979). Adolescent smoking: Onset and prevention. *Pediatrics, 63*, 650-658.

McAnarney, E. R., & Schreider, C. (1984). *Identifying social and psychological antecedents of adolescent pregnancy.* New York: William T. Grant Foundation.

Miller, P., & Simon, W. (1974). Adolescent sexual behavior: Context and changes. *Social Problems, 22*(1), 58-76.

Mindick, B., & Oskamp, S. (1979). Longitudinal predictive research: An approach to methodological problems in studying contraception. *Population and Environment, 2*(3), 259-276.

Mindick, B., & Oskamp, S. (1982). Individual differences among adolescent contraceptors: Some implications for intervention. In I. Stuart & C. Wells (Eds.), *Pregnancy in adolescence: Needs, problems and management* (pp. 140-176). New York: Van Nostrand Reinhold Co.

Moore, & Caldwell. (1977). *Out of wedlock childbearing.* Washington, DC: Urban Institute.

Nadelson, C. C., Hatman, M. T., & Gellon, J. W. (1980). Sexual knowledge and attitudes of adolescents: Relationship to contraceptive use. *Obstetrics and Gynecology, 55,* 340-345.

National Center for Health Statistics. (1978, March 29). Final natality statistics, 1976: Advance report. *Monthly Vital Statistics Report, 26*(12), 1-26. [DHEW Publication No. (PHS) 78-1120]

Olson, C. F., & Worsbey, J. (1984). Perceived mother-daughter relations in a pregnant and nonpregnant adolescent sample. *Adolescence, 119*(76), 781-794.

Olson, L. (1980). Social and psychological correlates of pregnancy resolution among adolescent women: A review. *American Journal of Orthopsychiatry, 50*(3), 432-445.

Perlman, S. B., Klerman, L. V., & Kinard, E. M. (1981). The use of socioeconomic data to predict teenage birth rates: An exploratory study in Massachusetts. *Public Health Reports, 96*(4), 335-341.

Pocs, D., Godow, A., Tolone, W., & Walsh, R. (1977). Is there sex after 40? *Psychology Today, 11*(1), 54-56, 87.

Quay, H. C. (1981). Psychological factors in teenage pregnancy. In K. G. Scott, T. Fields, & E. Robertson (Eds.), *Teenage parents and their offspring* (pp. 73-90). New York: Grune and Stratton.

Reid, D. (1982). School sex education and the causes of unintended teenage pregnancies: A review. *Health Education Journal, 41*(1), 4-11.

Rogel, M., & Zuehlke, M. (1982). Adolescent contraceptive behaviors: Influences and implications. In I. Stuart & C. Wells (Eds.), *Pregnancy in adolescence: Needs, problems and management* (pp. 194-218). New York: Van Nostrand Reinhold Company.

Rosen, R. H., & Ager, J. W. (1981). Self-concept and contraception: Pre-conception decision making. *Population and Environment, 4*(1), 11-23.

Rosenberg, P. B. (1980). Communication about sex and birth control between mothers and their adolescent children. *Population Environment, 3*(1), 35-50.

Rutter, M. (1980). *Changing youth in a changing society.* Cambridge, MA: Harvard University Press.

Sandberg, E. C., & Jacobs, R. I. (1971). Psychology of the misuse and rejection of contraception. *American Journal of Obstetrics and Gynecology, 110*(2), 227-242.

Scales, P. (1983). Adolescent sexuality and education: Principles, approaches, and resources. In C. S. Chilman (Ed.), *Adolescent sexuality in a changing American society* (pp. 207-229). New York: Wiley.

Scheirer, M. A. (1983). Household structure among welfare families: Correlates and consequences. *Journal of Marriage and the Family, 45*(4), 761-771.

Schinke, S. P. (1978). Teenage pregnancy: The need for multiple casework services. *Social Casework, 59*(7), 406-410.

Schinke, S. P. (1979). Research on adolescent health: Social work implications. In W. T. Hall & C. Y. Young (Eds.), *Health and social needs of the adolescent: Professional responsibilities* (pp. 320-351). Pittsburgh: University of Pittsburgh Graduate School of Public Health.

Schinke, S. P. (1982). School-based model for preventing teenage pregnancy. *Social Work in Education, 4*(2), 34-42.

Schinke, S. P. (1984). Preventing teenage pregnancy. In M. Hersen, P. Eisler, & P.

Miller (Eds.), *Progress in behavior modification* (Vol *16*, pp. 31-64). Orlando, FL: Academic.

Schinke, S. P., Blythe, B. J., Gilchrist, L. D., & Burt, G. A. (1981). Primary prevention of adolescent pregnancy. *Social Work With Groups, 4*(2), 121-135.

Schinke, S. P., & Gilchrist, L. D. (1977). Adolescent pregnancy: An interpersonal skill training approach to prevention. *Social Work in Health Care, 3*(2), 159-167.

Schinke, S. P., & Gilchrist, L. D. (1984). *Life skills counseling with adolescents.* Baltimore: University Park Press.

Schinke, S. P., Gilchrist, L. D., & Blythe, B. J. (1980). Role of communication in the prevention of teenage pregnancy. *Health and Social Work, 5,* 54-60.

Schinke, S. P., Gilchrist, L. D., & Small, R. W. (1979). Preventing unwanted adolescent pregnancy: A cognitive-behavioral approach. *American Journal of Orthopsychiatry, 49*(1), 81-88.

Septo, R., Keith, L., & Keith, D. (1975). Obstetrical and medical problems. In J. Zackler & W. Bradstadt (Eds.), *The teenage pregnant girl* (pp. 83-133). Springfield, IL: Charles C Thomas.

Sheehy, G. (1974). *Passages.* New York: E. P. Dutton & Co., Inc.

Smith, P. B., Weinman, M. L., & Mumford, D. M. (1982). Social and effective factors associated with adolescent pregnancy. *Journal of School Health, 52*(2), 90-93

Stiffman, A. R., & Morse, C. E. (1986). Adolescent sexuality, contraception, and pregnancy: Problems, programs and progress. *Practice Applications, 3*(2).

Thornburg, H. D. (1981). The amount of sex information learning obtained during early adolescence. *Journal of Early Adolescence, 1*(3), 171-183.

Toohey, J. V., & Valenzuela, G. J. (1982). Values clarification as a technique for family planning education. *Journal of School Health, 53*(2), 121-125.

Trussell, J., & Menken, J. (1978). Early childbearing and subsequent fertility. *Family Planning Perspectives, 10*(4), 209-218.

U. S. Bureau of the Census. *Households and family characteristics — March, 1983* (Series P-20, No. 388, Current Population Reports). Washington, DC: U. S. Government Printing Office.

Urburg, K. (1982). A theoretical framework for studying contraception use. *Adolescence, 17*(67), 527-540.

Ventura, S., & Hendershort, G. (1984). Infant health consequences of childbearing by teenagers and older mothers. *Public Health Reports, 99*(2), 138-146.

Wagner, N. (1970). Adolescent sexual behavior. In E. Evans (Ed.), *Adolescents: Readings in behavior and development.* Hinsdale, IL: Dryden Press.

Wodarski, J. S., Parham, T. M., Lindsey, E. W., & Blackburn, B. (1986). Reagan's AFDC policy changes: The Georgia experience. *Social Work, 31*(4), 273-279.

Yankelovich, Skelly, & White, Inc. (1979). *The General Mills American family report, 1978-79.* Minneapolis: General Mills.

Zelnik, M., & Kantner, J. (1977). Sexual and contraceptive experiences of young unmarried women in the U. S.: 1971-1976. *Family Planning Perspectives, 9*(2), 55-71.

Zelnik, M., & Kantner, J. (1979). Reasons for nonuse of contraception by sexually active women aged 15-19. *Family Planning Perspectives, 11,* 289-296.

Zelnik, M., & Kantner, J. (1980). Sexual activity, contraceptive use and pregnancy among metropolitan area teenagers: 1971-1979. *Family Planning Perspectives,*

12(5), 230.

Zelnik, M., & Kim, Y. J. (1982). Sex education and its association with teenage sexual activity, pregnancy, and contraceptive use. *Family Planning Perspectives, 14*(3), 117-126.

Zelnik, M., & Shah, F. (1983). First intercourse among young Americans. *Family Planning Perspectives, 15*(2), 64-70.

Chapter 5

ADOLESCENT SUBSTANCE ABUSE: PRACTICE IMPLICATIONS

A N ESTIMATED 18 million adults 18 years and older in the United States currently experience problems as a result of alcohol use. Of these, 10.6 million suffer from the disease of alcoholism. Alcohol-related problems may include symptoms of alcohol dependence such as memory loss, inability to stop drinking until intoxicated, inability to cut down on drinking, binge drinking, and withdrawal symptoms. Alcohol abuse and alcoholism cost the United States $116.8 billion in 1983. Costs due to premature death were $18 billion, reduced productivity cost $65.6 billion, and treatment cost $13.5 billion. Alcohol is a factor in nearly half of all accidental deaths, suicides and homicides, including 42 percent of all deaths from motor vehicle accidents. The intravenous drug user population (including homosexual IV drug users) accounts for 25 percent of all AIDS patients. The disease is contracted through sexual transmission and the sharing of contaminated needles among this group (National Institute on Drug Abuse, 1987).

Seventy million Americans, or 37 percent of the total U. S. population aged 12 and above, have used marijuana, cocaine, or another illicit drug at some time in their lives according to the most recent National Household Survey of Drug Abuse (National Institute on Drug Abuse, 1985). Twenty-three million, or 12 percent, were "current" users, i.e. they had used an illegal drug within the last 30 days. The use of marijuana and other drugs had declined since the comparable 1982 survey, although cocaine use increased.

Adolescence has been identified as a time when experimentation with drugs may be most active (Gorsuch & Arno, 1978; Mayer & Filstead,

1980). The acute consequences of substance use and misuse include traffic accidents, death due to accidents, later life health problems, suicide, school-related problems, temporary sickness, and absenteeism (Barr, Antes, Ottenberg, & Rosen, 1984). In addition, several studies have delineated the possible consequences of adolescent substance abuse which manifest themselves in antisocial behaviors (Gropper, 1984; Kane & Patterson, 1972; MacKay, 1961). Long-range consequences of teenage substance misuse include the failure to formulate goals for the future (Goodstadt & Sheppard, 1983) and stigmatization following an arrest while under the influence of drugs. The labeling of an adolescent under these circumstances can result in the loss of status, opportunity, and personal self-esteem (Mayer & Filstead, 1980). Patterns of substance abuse also have significant health consequences (Prendergast & Schafer, 1974).

The cost of drinking and subsequent driving among teenagers presents a significant social problem in this country. In 1980 alone there were 1,289,443 persons arrested for driving while under the influence of alcohol. Of those, 29,957 were under the age of 18 and 696 were under age 15! And there appears to be a trend toward a progressively worsening situation. Arrests for DUI among the 18 and under age group increased 236 percent between 1971 and 1980.

The outcomes of adolescent DUI are deadly. In one account, 43 percent of the approximately 50,000 persons killed in motor vehicle accidents were correlated with adolescent DUI (Alcohol Health and Research World, 1983). In an address at the NIAAA Alcohol and Drug Education Conference on October 4, 1982, former Health and Human Services Secretary Richard S. Schweiker stated that over 10,000 young people die in alcohol-related motor vehicle crashes each year (Allen, 1983, p. 4).

Current drug users among youth (12-17) are also polydrug users. Of those who smoke cigarettes, 74 percent also drink alcohol, 47 percent use marijuana, and 9 percent use cocaine. Among those who drink alcohol, 37 percent also use marijuana and 5 percent use cocaine. Among those who use marijuana, 60 percent smoke cigarettes, 84 percent drink alcohol, and 12 percent use cocaine (National Institute on Drug Abuse, 1985).

The statistics bear witness to the gravity of the problem. People of all ages are dying at an alarming rate from substance abuse. Yet, society's attitude towards drugs is one of ambivalence (West, Maxwell, Noble, &

Solomon, 1984). Macrosystem changes are called for in order to reorient society to the dangers of its complacency. Substance abuse is a problem for all age groups and for the total social system. The individual, his/her peer group, the family (both nuclear and extended), the school, and the community at large are all affected by the escapades of just one substance-abusing individual.

Attempts to reverse the trend of acceptance of substance abuse have been characterized by their focus on only certain aspects of the problem. This singular focus has resulted in limited effectiveness of prevention programs (Johnson, 1984; Wodarski & Hoffman, 1984).

Findings from the University of Michigan's Institute for Social Research's multi-year Monitoring the Future surveys ("Patterns of Drug Use," 1987-1988) continue to tell a troubling story of drug use among young people nationwide. Responses to the 1987 survey indicate that over half of last year's high school seniors (57%) had tried an illicit drug, and over one-third (36%) had tried an illicit drug other than marijuana. One in every six or seven high school seniors had tried cocaine (15.2%) and one in eighteen (5.6%) had tried "crack" — the especially risky form of cocaine. The study also reveals that by age 27, nearly 40 percent of young adults have had some experience with cocaine. Two other classes of drugs — alcohol and cigarettes — have remained overwhelmingly popular among young people. Nearly all of 1987s high school seniors (92%) reported some experience with alcohol, and nearly 40 percent reported having had five or more drinks in a row in the two weeks just prior to the survey.

Adolescence is a time when the relative importance of family and peers begins to shift. It is also viewed as a time of stress for both the adolescent and his/her family. Substance abuse, particularly for minority youths, is frequently a part of the stress experienced, as it may be either the cause or the effect (Petersen & Hamburg, 1986). As such, it is important to develop programs to prevent substance abuse. As school, peers, and family are the primary influences on an adolescent's life, preventive programs should focus on these three areas to increase their prosocial influences.

This chapter addresses the multiple forces impacting upon adolescents and resulting in substance abuse. The aim is to propose means by which to effect macro-level change in societal norms and values regarding substance abuse. There are a number of avenues through which change can be made. This chapter will explore the following subsystems as areas of change: (1) development of appropriate treatment paradigms, (2) school and peer group environments, (3) home and family, (4) media, (5) community movements, and (6) business and industry.

Effective Treatment Paradigms

If the field of substance abuse is to progress and effective treatment and prevention paradigms are to be developed, the causal nature of substance abuse must be identified. The role that biological, cognitive, and learning variables play in the development and maintenance of substance abuse behaviors must be ascertained. Once this knowledge is developed, specific paradigms can be formulated according to type of client, with what type of techniques, where, and how long. Moreover, this development should include follow-up studies to ascertain the maintenance of achieved therapeutic gains.

The causal nature of substance abuse, however, is complicated and multifaceted. Most likely, each facet will require unique conceptualization of the causal chain and structuring of appropriate strategies. For example, each one of the following paradigms could be developed: substance abuse among pregnant mothers, minorities, adolescents, and so forth. Until these knowledge bases are developed, means to reduce the effects of substance abuse will be minimal (Heather & Robertson, 1981).

SUBSTANCE ABUSE: THEORETICAL PERSPECTIVE

Adolescence is a time when individuals become more oriented toward their peers and less toward their parents (Botvin, 1983; Bronfenbrenner, 1974; Montemayor, 1982). Adolescents turn to peers in order to receive emotional support that inattentive and unconcerned parents fail to provide. Hill (1980) stresses the importance of the conflict between parent and adolescent which leads to the adolescent accepting or seeking the approval of peers. Substantial data are available to indicate that, relative to the pre-adolescent years, parents and adolescent perceptions of conflict increase, actual conflict increases, and effective communication decreases between parents and adolescents (e.g. Montemayor, 1982; Smith & Forehand, in press). Simultaneously, peers become increasingly influential (Montemayor, 1982). Therefore, the relative importance of family and peers must be carefully considered in adolescent drug prevention programs. As Glynn (1981) has indicated, theoretical approaches to this issue range from those which view either family (Hirschi, 1969) or peers (Sutherland & Cressey, 1970) as the primary influence to those which view both family and peers as important but typically in different domains of behavior (e.g. Kandel, Kessler, & Margulies, 1978; Pentz, 1983).

Adolescence is a critical period for the development of social, cognitive, and academic skills. It is essential that we identify appropriate intervention foci to decrease substance abuse during this developmental period. At present, the best model for viewing family and peer influence on adolescent drug use is one developed by Kandel and her colleagues (e.g. Kandel, 1974a, 1974b, 1981; Kandel & Faust, 1975; Kandel et al., 1978). Among other influences, the influence of parents and peers on each of the following three stages of drug use is considered: (1) initiation to hard liquor, (2) then marijuana, and finally (3) other illicit drugs. Based on a review of the available research, Glynn (1981) concludes that parents are most influential in adolescent initiation into hard liquor use and in adolescent initiation into use of illicit drugs other than marijuana, whereas peers are the primary influence in marijuana use. Parental modeling of drug use and the parental relationship with his/her adolescent are the primary mechanisms identified in adolescent drug use, whereas modeling alone appears to be the primary mechanism for peer influence.

Our theoretical perspective, as is Kandel's, is anchored within a broad base of social learning theory (Robin & Foster, 1984). From this viewpoint, the adolescent learns appropriate and inappropriate behavior from the context (that is, parents and peers) in which he/she functions by modeling and reinforcement (Bandura, 1969). That is, by observing the behaviors demonstrated by others and by receiving or not receiving reinforcement/punishment for engaging in such behaviors, adolescents acquire certain behavior patterns. Furthermore, and of particular importance, if an adolescent functions within a context in which good communication and/or adequate cognitive skills are lacking [e.g. he/she has inadequate knowledge and unrealistic beliefs, expectations or attributions (Robin & Foster, 1984)], he/she is more likely to engage in maladaptive behavior patterns through modeling and reinforcement. Such a developmental process does not provide the adolescent with the requisite behaviors for prosocial attachment to family members, peers, and social institutions and is a high-risk factor for subsequent substance abuse.

While researchers are increasing their data base about teenage substance abuse and its consequences and are beginning to develop theoretical models of drug abuse, they know little about the effective prevention of substance misuse among teenagers. The solution to the problem of adolescent substance abuse among teens will require an all-out effort by families, schools, peers and communities (Fors & Rojeck, 1983; Wodarski & Fisher, 1986). However, to this point most programs have focused on only one of these variables (for reviews see Dembo & Burgos, 1976; Gullotta & Adams, 1982; Janvier, Guthman, & Catalano, 1980; Kinder, Pape, & Walfish, 1980; Schinke & Gilchrist, 1985).

As peers and parents are the best predictors of adolescent drug use (Adler & Kandel, 1982; Glynn, 1981), preventive programs are needed that include one or ideally both of these groups. Data now are emerging to suggest effective procedures for dealing with peers and parents in order to prevent substance abuse. Critical questions that must be addressed are the type of interventions, their subsequent foci, and how interventions differentially affect minority, non-minority, female and male adolescents.

A unique adolescent education program, Teams-Games-Tournaments (TGT), has been developed for use by school professionals to teach adolescents about alcohol to prevent its misuse. TGT was developed through extensive research on games used as teaching devices, using small groups as classroom work units, and emphasizing the task-and-reward structures used in the traditional classroom. The TGT technique is an alternative teaching approach that fully utilizes structure emphasizing group, rather than individual, achievement and utilizes peers as teachers and supporters of prosocial norms (Feldman & Wodarski, 1975; Wodarski, 1981; Wodarski et al., 1980). Thus, the TGT method capitalizes on peer influence, subsequently increases social attachment to peers which research suggests are major influencing factors in an adolescent's life, and influences the acquisition and subsequent maintenance of knowledge and behavior change.

Recent results of a large-scale study by Wodarski (1987a, 1987b, 1987c, 1988) support the effectiveness of TGT as a prevention strategy for alcohol abuse. In a study involving five school systems, high school students participated in a four-week educational program that focused on alcohol information and the application of the concepts to their own lives. The program emphasized behavioral objectives attained through self-management skills that lead to responsible drinking practices.

Included in the study were three groups: students receiving the TGT method, those receiving traditional instruction, and those receiving no instruction. A total of 1,400 subjects participated. The results indicated that the TGT method was superior to the remaining groups in terms of each of the following self-report measures: alcohol knowledge, reduction in drinking behavior, positive changes concerning drinking and driving, reduced impulsivity, and improvement in several self-concept measures. In addition, both teacher and student evaluations indicated that the TGT program was viewed as a positive and productive experience. A one- and two-year follow-up indicates all of the effects of the TGT method on knowledge and attitudes were maintained (Wodarski, 1987b, 1987c). Based on these positive results and other data, it would appear that TGT programs could be used for drug, as well as for alcohol, prevention programs and is the most effective method for altering a peer support system which, in many instances, supports drug usage.

The other significant variable that influences an adolescent's drug use is the family. In particular, parents serve as models in drug and alcohol use (Kandel, 1980); that is, the probability of drug experimentation and use is increased when adolescents view parents exhibiting such behaviors. Furthermore, particular types of parenting behavior (lack of positive reinforcement, setting appropriate expectations, communication skills, and problem-solving skills) can serve as predictors of adolescent drug use (Pulkkinen, 1983) and can discriminate between adolescent drug users and non-users (Rees & Wilborn, 1983). Therefore, it would appear that teaching parents to provide appropriate models and expectations, and improving parents' problem-solving and communication skills, would be critical ingredients of an adolescent drug prevention program for parents.

Basically, problem solving involves four steps: problem identification, generation of alternative solutions, decision making, and planning solution implementation (Robin & Foster, 1984). Communication involves skills which can be used during problem-solving discussions and at other times. Robin and Foster (1984) have identified 20 behaviors that may interfere with effective communication. These include accusing, putting down, interrupting, getting off topics, dwelling on the past, and threatening. Robin, Foster and their colleagues have conducted three well-controlled studies which support the effectiveness of a problem-solving communication skills training program for parents. Relative to waiting list control groups and a family therapy approach, problem-solving communication skills increase communication and decrease conflicts (Foster, Prinz, & O'Leary, 1983; Robin, 1981; Robin, Kent, O'Leary, Foster, & Prinz, 1977). Furthermore, at follow-ups improvements achieved with problem-solving skills were maintained.

If parents and peers are primary influences on adolescent drug use (e.g. Adler & Kandel, 1982; Glynn, 1981; Lewis & Lewis, 1984), then prevention efforts should be directed toward developing and systematically evaluating programs with these two groups. As indicated in the preceding paragraphs, data are available to suggest basic components for such programs.

School and Peer Group Environments

Youth spend the majority of their lives in the school setting. The school system, therefore, seems to be a natural forum for implementation of change. Educational programs aimed at prevention and early intervention can negate the powerful influence of peers.

An awareness of the problem of drug use among youth and recognition of ways in which society condones it are steps toward positive change. The schools can be instrumental in educating both the adolescents and their parents. Parents must be knowledgeable of the symptoms of substance abuse in adolescents. The usual signs of possible drug problems are radical changes in the usual behavioral patterns. "A definite drop in grades, bad conduct and skipping school" are typical according to Pat Schult, senior counselor for the Young Adult Teen on the Alcohol Detoxification Unit at Peachford Hospital, Atlanta, Georgia (Okel, 1984).

Substance use by teens takes its toll in other ways, also. The drug-abusing teen may feel isolated from non-abusing peers. Crime may become a factor to deal with when the adolescent has to steal to maintain drug habits. There are also developmental issues to be recognized. Adolescents already dealing with stressful changes in their lives may compound the stress with drug use. They are changing in physical, emotional and sexual ways and must deal with new roles, feelings and identities.

The issue is further compounded by multiple abuse patterns. Young people frequently use alcohol in combination with other drugs, principally marijuana (Lowman et al., 1982; Turanski, 1983). This combination of alcohol and drugs adds to the difficulty in treating youths and their changing values.

Junior and senior high schools can offer parents an educational and helping network using the school as a meeting place. One school developed such a network through a parent group that initially served in an informational capacity and subsequently as a resource and support group (Turanski, 1983).

Swisher (1976) suggests that programs addressing education and prevention should include "all activities which are *planned* to enrich the personal development of the student...including humanistic education, open education, affective education, values clarification, career education and developmental guidance." This is an all-encompassing approach which needs also to be reinforced in the other areas of youths' lives.

The ideal program should have two foci. First, the information transmission approach to provide basic knowledge and awareness, and second, the responsible decision approach that will teach youngsters the basic coping and decision-making skills (Schinke & Gilchrist, 1984).

It is important to remember that experimentation with drugs and peer pressure are related, and that peer pressure will be applied most dramatically in the school. Educators must aim to make teens more self-confident and less influenced by peer pressure. Globetti (1977) states that "in American society parents and peers are the primary socializing agencies in the onset and emergence of teenage attitudes and behavior regarding alcohol" (p. 167).

Programs must take advantage of peer pressure in a positive manner. To be non-judgmental and to develop self-esteem in these vulnerable youths are goals of utmost importance and urgency. In program planning there is a need for youth to provide input regarding what they feel are their greatest stresses and programs needed to directly address these issues.

Many youths use drugs as a coping mechanism. School pressures and adolescent growth (both emotional and physical) are all basic life problems. The schools can offer meaningful alternatives to drug use to help adolescents deal with these stressors. A variety of activities can be offered by schools to provide reinforcements for teenagers other than drugs. These after-school programs will be successful when they center on the youths' interests such as music, fashion, sports and so forth. For example, gyms can be kept open on weekends and during summer months, a small price compared to the cost of consequences of drugs.

The problem in reaching these adolescents comes when they do not see their drug use as a problem but as a regular boredom-relieving activity. When drug-using youth are asked if they see their drug use as a problem, the most frequently encountered reply is no (Turanski, 1983). When they do recognize a problem, youth are ill-prepared to seek help. They are more often than not unaware of drug prevention and treatment centers. Moreover, they may view these services with mistrust, fear and embarrassment. Another great fear is exposure to both parents and the law. Thus, communication has to occur regarding services that are available. Service providers have to reach out to the youths who are at risk.

Teams-Games-Tournaments Intervention

Adolescents participate in a six-week educational program focused on the understanding of drug information and the application of concepts to their own lives. The program emphasizes behavioral objectives aimed at acquisition of self-management skills.

The completion of the assessment of drug knowledge provides the basis for dividing students into four-member teams. The teams are organized into high achievers (those with a high level of drug knowledge), middle achievers (those with moderate levels), and low achievers (those most lacking in drug knowledge). The composition of the teams are heterogeneous, including one high achiever, two middle achievers, and one low achiever. Thus, the average achievement level is approximately equal across teams. The achievement levels of individual students on the assessment of drug knowledge is not revealed.

The drug education units contained in the curriculum guide are presented for fifty minutes each day for six weeks. The first three days of each week are devoted to learning drug concepts by discussions and various participatory activities. The fourth day focuses on working in the TGT teams on worksheets, in preparation for the tournament to be held on the fifth day of each week.

The tournament games consist of short-answer questions designed to reinforce and assess the knowledge gained in class. These are played by team members individually competing against other team members of comparable achievement levels. The team members are assigned to a tournament table, competing against two students of comparable achievement levels from other teams. Scores are kept for each individual during the tournament games. At the end of the tournament, the top, middle, and low scorers at each table are awarded a fixed number of points for their teams. The points earned determine whether a student will stay at the same tournament table or move to a table with higher or lower performing students for the next tournament. In this way competitors change regularly, and the competition is not skewed in favor of any group of achievers. The points earned by an individual are added to those earned by other team members to compose a total team score. Teachers tabulate team scores at the end of each tournament, and scores are posted on the next school day.

The special timeliness of TGT to teach adolescents about drugs and how to make better decisions regarding its usage is that when TGT is used, all students have an equal opportunity to succeed, because all students compete against members of other teams who are of similar achievement levels, and points earned by low achievers are just as valuable to the overall team score as points earned by high achievers. This is in contrast to the typical instructional method which centers on individual assessment compared to the total class. Thus, relative to individual instruction, the TGT method helps one of the high-risk populations for substance abuse (i.e. the low achieving student) to acquire knowledge (Newcomb, Maddahian, & Bentler, 1986). Moreover, there is significance in using the group reward structure with adolescents, in that it capitalizes on peer influence and reinforcement, which is considered to be one of the most potent variables in the acquisition, alteration, and maintenance of behavior in youth (Buckholdt & Wodarski, 1978).

The program of comprehensive drug education is comprised of the following components.

A. Drug Education

(1) **Biological, psychological, and sociocultural determinants of drug abuse.** It is crucial that in learning about drugs, participants become informed of the multiple factors that have been shown to contribute to irresponsible use of drugs and to dependence. This will serve to assist participants in making realistic judgments about their own present or possible future drug use, and to inform them of the progression of drug use from responsible, to problem usage, to dependence. Adolescents have been found to lack such knowledge (Kaplan, Martin, & Robbins, 1984).

(2) **Basic knowledge about drug consumption and usage.** Students learn the gamut of topics related to drug use, such as how much drugs can a body absorb in a given length of time, when an intoxicated person

is in an emergency situation and how to deal with such an occurrence, the physiological attributes of drugs in relation to the human body, the amount of alcohol in a variety of alcoholic beverages, and how to assess a drug problem.

(3) **Curriculum.**
(a) Drugs and Our Society
(b) What Are Drugs?
(c) Short-Term Effects of Drugs: Intoxication and Hangover
(d) Values Clarification and Drugs
(e) Common Motivations for Drug and Drug Behavior
(f) Long-Term Effects of Drugs
(g) Drugs and the Effects on Driving
(h) Alternatives to Drugs in Our Society
(i) Recognizing and Treating Drug Problems

Both areas, determinants of drug abuse and basic knowledge, are taught via group discussion, participatory activities, and the TGT tournaments, all emphasizing the use of peer support to enhance learning and the acceptance of responsible attitudes toward drugs.

B. Self-Management and Maintenance

Students are taught basic principles of social learning theory related to drug consumption from a self-management of life perspective. Social learning theory oriented psychologists emphasize that the abuse of drugs is learned from the consequences that follow. These most often include: (1) stress reduction (the reinforcer might be lessened inhibition in sociability around peers); (2) removal from an unpleasant situation (given that adolescents tend to abuse more at one sitting than adults, this behavior more often results in their passing out to deal with an unpleasant situation); and (3) an excuse for otherwise unacceptable behavior (the person being unusually aggressive or flirtatious could be excused on the basis of being intoxicated).

Other potential reinforcers for drug abuse are in abundance: modeling peer drug use in order to gain acceptance, peer pressure to drink or take drugs and subsequent reinforcement by significant peers, having fun equated with how much one drinks, and the need to escape from thought of academic failure.

A fundamental theme students learn is that one can change or determine behavior by altering one's environment and thus developing different options for rewards. This may be the internal environment or the external environment. The two major categories of environmental events which must be understood and manipulated to produce the desired outcome are events which precede and set the stage for particular behaviors, and events which follow the behavior and make them more or less likely to occur (Williams & Long, 1979). Thus, one task of the learning experience of the proposed program is to help students identify environmental events controlling behavior and to alter the ones necessary to produce the desired behavior.

Examples of external environmental stimuli which cue substance abuse behaviors are parties or peer modeling of drug use. Examples of internal environmental events are emotional upset and loneliness. Students are instructed in how to remove or reduce stress-producing cues, such as irrational beliefs and faulty assessment of others' behavior, from the environment and how to engage in rewarding activities other than the consumption of drugs (Botvin, Baker, Botvin, Filazzola, & Millman, 1984).

A necessary aspect of self-management particularly pertinent to drugs and their use is learning to be assertive with others (Horan & Williams, 1982). Recent research has shown that young-adult problem drug abusers often feel dissatisfaction with their interpersonal relationships with others and perceive themselves as lacking in social skills.

The adolescent learns how to better cope with the task of interacting with others in a meaningful and satisfying way. Facets of this program developed by Lange and Jakubowski (1976) are used. These involve conversational skills training, use of appropriate non-verbal communication, and development of assertive behavior in learning to decrease stress produced by inadequately met social needs.

Specific elements emphasized are how to: introduce oneself, initiate and continue conversations, give and receive compliments, enhance appearance, make and refuse requests, express feelings spontaneously, use appropriate non-verbal behavior in enhancing sociability with others, reward oneself for not drinking or taking drugs, and discuss alternatives for help with a significant other with a drinking or drug problem. Role-play simulation exercises are used to help adolescents practice how to refuse drugs in a socially acceptable manner within normal peer contexts. This aspect of the program is modeled after the work of Foy, Miller, Eisler, and O'Toole (1976). General procedures are referred to as drink/drug refusal training. The basic aim is to help students develop more effective ways of dealing with social pressures to consume drugs.

Specific situations are practiced where individuals apply pressure to persuade others to consume excessive amounts of drugs. Students practice reactions to statements like: "One drink and/or pill won't hurt you," "What kind of friend are you?" or "Just have a little one, I'll make sure you won't have any more."

These areas of self-management skills are taught through group discussion and participatory activities and, where appropriate, are incorporated into the TGT tournaments.

Adolescents also need training in terms of coping with the daily problems of living, i.e. their academic and social concerns. They are taught a problem-solving approach based on the work of Robin and Foster (1984).

The general components emphasized are:

(1) problem definition
(2) how to generate possible solutions
(3) decision making
(4) how to choose and implement strategies through the following procedures:
    a. general introduction to how the provision of certain consequences and stimuli can control problem-solving behavior
    b. isolation and definition of a behavior to be changed
    c. use of stimulus control techniques to influence rates of problem-solving behavior
    d. use of appropriate consequences to either increase or decrease a behavior
(5) verification of the outcome and renegotiation.

The Family

That "kids will learn what you tell them about drinking" is a myth that must be dispelled according to the United States Jaycee's Operation THRESHOLD pamphlet, "Drinking Myths." The fact is that "your kids will learn what you show them about drinking. If you drink heavily; if you get drunk; the chances are your kids will follow the same example." Thus, the mandate is clear that parents must set examples for their children.

Young people need positive role models from which to gain their experiences. Data indicate that adolescents are more likely to consume drugs in a manner similar to that of their parents (Wodarski & Hoffman, 1984) and the parents' drug behavior is an important influence (Bacon & Jones, 1968).

Drinking is frequently associated with "coming of age" (Pittman & Snyder, 1962), and a driver's license and the availability of alcohol are symbols of adulthood. While forming their new identities, teens need "adult clarification and support in their process of becoming independent" (Lieberman, Caroff, & Gottesfeld, 1973).

The family is the "crucial influence on children's values and behavior" (Lieberman et al., 1973). In the home, youth can find structure and guidance from loved ones who really care about them. Clear expectations about consumption can be communicated. Younger children are especially vulnerable to pressures and they need a trusting and comfortable place to turn for help in mastering their anxieties and frustrations. The home is the stabilizing influence for youth. It should be the place to turn where drug-induced states are not glorified.

Parents must realize that in regard to drugs and driving they maintain ultimate control. Parents are the resource for the car availability. Mom and dad have the power to keep the car from abusing adolescents. Parents need to be reinforced that they have the responsibility and right to make decisions that are in the best interests of their children.

Parents may need help in asserting themselves and in coping with difficult situations. Support is available through such mechanisms as Parent Effectiveness Training (PET) classes where parents learn better parenting skills. Through such training, parents learn to set clear expectations about drugs and to enforce consequences when expectations are not met. Moreover, they practice ways to open lines of communication to discuss the use of drugs and their effects with their teenager.

Family Prevention Strategy

Parents participate in a five-week program in which they will meet in groups of 10 families (both parents, if possible) two hours each week. Like the TGT procedures, the initial focus is on learning drug concepts. This information is dispensed in handouts and is discussed within the first two-hour group session. Topics covered include how much drugs the body can absorb in a given length of time, when an intoxicated person is in an emergency situation and how to deal with such an occurrence, the physiological attributes of drugs in relation to the human body, the amount of alcohol in various alcoholic beverages, and how to assess a drug problem. Also, long- and short-term effects of drugs and various types of drugs that are available are covered.

During the second session basic knowledge about drug consumption and usage is continued from the first session. Variables that initiate and maintain drug usage are covered. In addition, data on parent use of drugs and its effects on adolescents' drug use is elaborated.

The third and fourth sessions are devoted to teaching problem-solving skills and communication skills for conflict resolution (Robin & Foster, 1984). The five steps involved in problem solving are delineated: problem definition, generation of alternate solutions, decision making, planning solution implementation, and renegotiation. Based on Robin and Foster (1984) parents are initially presented with these steps in the following way. Ideas are presented in lecture form and then discussed in the group, and then role playing of how to use the procedures are implemented. The role playing consists of selected group members attempting to solve problems of adolescents of other group members.

When the basic steps for problem-solving have been delineated and practiced, communication training is implemented with particular emphasis on listening carefully, using reflective statements, reaching agreements before terminating a discussion, and using contracts. The communication targets (Robin & Foster, 1984) listed in Table 5-1 will be distributed to parents. The various problematic behaviors are discussed as well as the possible alternatives. Presentation of problematic and appropriate behavior is conducted by group leaders. Subsequently, various participants role-play problem-solving situations and receive feedback from other group members concerning their use of communication/conflict resolution skills.

In sessions three and four, information is delineated on use of positive and negative control with adolescents. The focus within this material is on increasing use of positive reinforcement for appropriate behavior rather than often used coercive processes such as negative reinforcement and punishment (Forehand & McMahon, 1981; Patterson, 1981).

In the fifth session, the use of problem-solving, communication training and positive reinforcement procedures are integrated and applied to drug and alcohol prevention. It is emphasized that generally using communication skills, problem-solving skills, and positive reinforcement will result in a better relationship with their adolescents (better communication, less conflict) and, therefore, reduce the probability of drug and alcohol use. However, it is also emphasized that these skills can be utilized directly in order to discuss drug and alcohol use and to implement solutions if drug and alcohol use is occurring.

Table 5-1

DICTIONARY OF COMMUNICATION TARGETS

Problematic Behavior	*Possible Alternative*
1. Talking through a third person.	Talking directly to another person.
2. Accusing, blaming, defensive statements.	Making I-statements (I feel _____ when _____ happens).
3. Putting down, zapping, shaming.	Accepting responsibility, I-statement.
4. Interrupting (other than for clarification).	Listening; raising hand or gesturing when wanting to talk. Encouraging speakers to use brief statements.
5. Overgeneralizing, catastrophizing, making extremist, rigid statements.	Qualifying, making tentative statements (sometimes, maybe, etc.); accurate quantitative statements.
6. Lecturing, preaching, moralizing	Making brief, explicit problem statements (I would like _____).
7. Talking in a sarcastic tone of voice.	Talking in a neutral tone of voice.
8. Failing to make eye contact.	Looking at the person with whom you are talking.
9. Fidgeting, moving restlessly, or gesturing while being spoken to.	Sitting in a relaxed fashion. Excusing self for being restless.
10. Mindreading (attributing thoughts and feelings to another without the other's having communicated these feelings).	Reflecting, paraphrasing, validating.
11. Getting off the topic.	Catching self and returning to the problem as defined.
12. Commanding, ordering.	Suggesting alternative solutions.
13. Dwelling on the past.	Sticking to the present and future, suggesting changes to correct past problems.
14. Monopolizing the conversation.	Taking turns, making brief statements.
15. Intellectualizing, pedanticizing.	Speaking in simple, clear language that a teenager can understand.
16. Threatening.	Suggesting alternative solutions.
17. Humoring, discounting.	Reflecting, validating.
18. Incongruence between verbal and non-verbal behavior.	Matching verbal affect and non-verbal posture.

Media

The media exert a powerful influence on contemporary society. Examples of both positive and negative portrayals of substance abuse behavior in terms of setting appropriate expectations for drug consumption are aired throughout the viewing period. Depending on the programming, the messages are as varied as "drinking is mandated for a good time" and "to be a good friend, do not let your friend drink and drive." Young people "watch television and see the message of what they need and what they should want. 'Tuning in can lead to turning off by turning on' " (Lieberman et al., 1973, p. 110). Also, as Globetti (1977) suggests, "Adolescents...view drugs mostly in terms of sociability and in the sense of what it does *for* them rather than *to* them."

The significant impact of daytime and nighttime TV "soaps" needs to be evaluated. Such programs as "Dallas" need parents' interpretation. Excessive consumption as portrayed in these shows is equated with power and success. In reality, adolescents must be informed that such consumption more likely impedes success.

The media can likewise exert a powerful positive influence. One of the favorite pasttimes of contemporary youth is music. The messages this media conveys must be considered since it is a continual influence. The biggest name in music today is Michael Jackson. Children of all ages have heard him on the radio and have seen him in magazines and newspapers. This young man has had a significant positive influence on youth. His million-dollar recording of "Beat It" has been rewritten to address substance abuse. Because of his commitment to youth, the White House has recognized him with a special plaque and reception hosted by President Reagan (ABC News Announcement, 1984). Positive role models such as Jackson affect the norms of youth and must be capitalized upon. Rather than glorify the consumption of drugs and its association with adventure and sex, role models can "turn on" teens to more positive outlets.

Community Movements

The ability to influence community norms rests within the community itself. By joining forces and establishing coalitions, standards of acceptance of substance abuse can be changed (Blansfield, 1984; Gardner, 1983).

Locally sponsored "Soberfests" have provided education and awareness about the impact of irresponsible drug use on society. In some communities, these events are sponsored by a coalition of "business, voluntary organizations, churches and synagogues, universities, tax-supported agencies, hospitals and medical facilities, civic organizations and others who have community wellness and a positive, aggressive, innovative approach to health " as a primary goal. They promote "new norms...stay alive; don't drink and drive; get high on life; and, it's OK not to drink" (Athens Community Wellness Council, 1984). Community-wide campaigns promote awareness of behaviors that "add enjoyment and years to life" and are a positive influence on community norms.

Other community organizations, such as the United States Jaycees with the Operation THRESHOLD, have taken steps to offer responsible alternatives to the norms that allow irresponsible drinking and driving under the influence (1983). Mothers Against Drunk Driving (MADD) is a grassroots organization that has succeeded in getting legislation passed for more adequate laws and enforcement. Such groups also provide social support necessary to sustain the work involved in such endeavors (Linblad, 1983).

Laws and Enforcement

Individual and community involvement and pressure can result in significant social change through governmental legislation and policy. On July 17, 1984, President Reagan signed into law a bill reducing federal highway aid to states that refuse to raise the legal drinking age to 21 by the year 1986. This law also provides extra funding to states that penalize drunken drivers with automatic jail sentences and revoked licenses (Atlanta Journal, July 18, 1984). He changed his original stance on this issue after becoming aware that states that have raised their drinking age have seen a drop in alcohol-related accidents. Government officials, grassroots organizations and private citizens provided the necessary push to get the legislation passed. With this new law comes a clear, though long overdue, message to today's youth: Drinking and driving is a problem that requires social action. Stronger enforcement of drug laws with absolute penalties is vital, with our government becoming more involved with source country crop control, interdiction efforts aimed at stopping illicit drugs at our border, and street-level enforcement through the use of physical surveillance or "buy and bust" operations (Moore, 1988).

Business and Industry

Business and industry have shown concern about substance abuse. They have been spurred to action by data that indicate that productivity is substantially reduced when workers abuse substances (Mayer, 1983). Moreover, they are recognizing that work is a central aspect in many lives and that supportive business can foster positive attitudes concerning the consumption of substances. Their commitment has been expressed by repeated advertisements in the media. They are reaching a large number of markets through use of printed media, such as advertisements in major magazines. Business-sponsored radio and television spots also promote responsible drinking. These spots have been used especially during holiday periods when people of all ages celebrate by irresponsibly using alcohol.

A General Motors advertisement that explains blood alcohol concentrations begins with a disclaimer: "First, you should understand that drinking any amount of alcohol can impair your ability to drive" (General Motors, 1983). The advertisement copy goes on to explain that General Motors has developed a device to test drivers' reflexes and responses before it allows the car to start. The Department of Transportation in California is now testing the device as a deterrent to repeat offenders. General Motors has made other commitments. For example, it set up a program for alcohol abuse in 1972 *(Newsweek,* August 22, 1983) and it has expanded its Employee Assistance Program to include every General Motors installation in the United States and 12 that are located in Canada.

CONCLUSION

The solution to the problem of substance abuse requires an all-out effort by those societal forces capable of effecting change. Families, schools, peers, communities, businesses and the media all possess powers to eradicate this social problem. The campaign cannot be waged from only one front, however. Combined cooperative efforts are essential. The responsibility must be shared for both previous condoning of actions that have perpetuated the problem and for working toward mutual goals and solutions.

The incidence of adolescent substance abuse and practice limitations have been reviewed. Variables that might be altered to prevent abuse among clients have been discussed. The chapter reviewed the following: effective treatment paradigms, school and peer environment, home and family, community movements, and business and industry in terms of how they can be employed to prevent substance abuse. The chapter concluded with an elucidation of what must be done to reduce adolescent substance abuse in America.

REFERENCES

ABC News Announcement, May 10, 1984.

Adler, I., & Kandel, D. B. (1982). A cross-cultural comparison of sociopsychological factors in alcohol use among adolescents in Israel, France, and the United States. *Journal of Youth and Adolescence, 11,* 89-113.

Alcohol Health and Research World. (March 3, 1983).

Allen, T. J. (1983). The school as a family suport system. *The U. S. Journal of Drug and Alcohol Dependence, 6*(3), 4.

Athens Community Wellness Council. (1984). *Up with wellness.* Athens, GA: Author.

Atlanta Journal. (July 18, 1984).

Bacon, M., & Jones, M. B. (1968). *Teenage drinking.* New York: Thomas Y. Crowell Company.

Bandura, A. (1969). *Principles of behavior modification.* New York: Holt, Rinehart & Winston.

Barr, H., Antes, D., Ottenberg, D., & Rosen, A. (1984). The mortality of treated alcoholics and drug addicts: The benefits of sobriety. *Journal of Studies on Alcohol, 45*(5), 440-452.

Blansfield, H. N. (1984). Drinking and/or driving. *Connecticut Medicine, 48*(3), 205.

Botvin, G. J. (1983). Prevention of adolescent substance abuse through the development of personal and social competence. In *Preventing adolescent drug abuse: Intervention strategies* [DHHS Publication No. (ADM) 83-1280]. Washington, DC: U. S. Government Printing Office.

Botvin, G. J., Baker, E., Botvin, E. M., Filazzola, A. D., & Millman, R. B. (1984). Prevention of alcohol misuse through the development of personal and social competence: A pilot study. *Journal of Studies on Alcohol, 45*(6), 550-552.

Bronfenbrenner, U. (1974). The origins of alienation. *Scientific American, 231,* 53-61.

Buckholdt, D., & Wodarski, J. S. (1978). The effects of different reinforcement systems on cooperative behavior exhibited by children in classroom contexts. *Journal of Research and Development in Education, 12*(1), 50-68.

Dembo, R., & Burgos, W. (1976). A framework for developing drug abuse prevention strategies for young people in ghetto areas. *Journal of Drug Education, 6*(4), 313-325.

Feldman, R. A., & Wodarski, J. S. (1975). *Contemporary approaches to group treatment.* San Francisco: Jossey-Bass.

Forehand, R., & McMahon, R. J. (1981). *Helping the non-compliant child: A clinician's guide to parent training.* New York: Guilford.

Fors, S. W., & Rojek, D. G. (1983). The social and demographic correlates of adolescent drug use patterns. *Journal of Drug Education, 13,* 205-222.

Foster, S. L., Prinz, R. J., & O'Leary, K. D. (1983). Impact of problem-solving communication training and generalization procedures on family conflict. *Child and Family Behavior Therapy, 5,* 1-24.

Foy, C. W., Miller, P. M., Eisler, R. M., & O'Toole, O. H. (1976). Social skills training to teach alcoholics to refuse drinks effectively. *Journal of Studies on Alcohol, 37*(9), 1340-1345.

Gardner, S. E. (1983). *Communities: What you can do about drug and alcohol abuse* (DHHS Pub. No. ADM-84-1310). Rockville, MD: National Institute on Drug Abuse.

General Motors. (1983, July). Customer information from General Motors. *GEO*, p. 5 (advertisement)

Globetti, G. (1977). Teenage drinking. In N. J. Estes & M. E. Heinemann (Eds.), *Alcoholism: Development, consequences and interventions.* St. Louis, MO: C. V. Mosby Co.

Glynn, T. J. (1981). From family to peer: A review of transitions of influence among drug-using youth. *Journal of Youth and Adolescence, 10,* 363-383.

Goodstadt, M. S., & Sheppard, M. A. (1983). Three approaches to alcohol education. *Journal of Studies on Alcohol, 44*(2), 362-380.

Gorsuch, R. L., & Arno, D. H. (1978). The relationship of children's attitudes toward alcohol to their value development. *Journal of Abnormal Child Psychology, 7*(31), 287-295.

Gropper, B. A. (1984). Probing the links between drugs and crime. *National Institute of Justice,* November, 4-8.

Gullotta, T., & Adams, G. R. (1982). Substance and youth programs. *Journal of Youth and Adolescence, 11,* 409-423.

Heather, N., & Robertson, I. (1981). *Controlled drinking.* New York: Methuen & Co.

Hill, J. P. (1980). The family. In M. Johnson (Ed.), *Toward adolescence: The middle school years.* Chicago: University of Chicago Press.

Hirschi, T. (1969). *Causes of delinquency.* Berkeley: University of California Press.

Horan, J. J., & Williams, J. M. (1982). Longitudinal study of assertion training as a drug abuse prevention strategy. *American Educational Research Journal, 19*(3), 341-351.

Janvier, R. L., Guthman, D. R., & Catalano, R. F. (1980). *An assessment of evaluation of drug abuse prevention programs.* Washington, DC: U. S. Superintendent of Documents, National Institute of Juvenile Justice and Delinquency Prevention.

Johnson, N. (1984). Research reports: Reducing community alcohol problems. *Alcohol Health and Research World, 8*(3), 60-61.

Kandel, D. (1974a). Inter- and intra-generational influences on adolescent marijuana use. *Journal of Social Issues, 30,* 107-135.

Kandel, D. (1974b). Interpersonal influences on adolescent drug use. In E. Josephson & E. Carroll (Eds.), *Drug use: Epidemiological and sociological approaches.* Washington, DC: Hemisphere.

Kandel, D. (1980). Developmental stages in adolescent drug involvement. In D. Lettieri (Ed.), *Theories of drug abuse* [DHHS Publication No. (ADM) 80-967]. Washington, DC: U. S. Government Printing Office.

Kandel, D. (1981). Adolescent marijuana use: Role of parents and peers. *Science, 181,* 1067-1070.

Kandel, D., & Faust, R. (1975). Sequences and stages in patterns of adolescent drug use. *Archives of General Psychiatry, 32,* 923-932.

Kandel, D., Kessler, R., & Margulies, R. (1978). Adolescent initiation into stages of drug use: A developmental analysis. In D. Kandel (Ed.), *Longitudinal research on drug use: Empirical findings on methodological issues.* Washington, DC: Hemisphere-Wiley.

Kane, R. L., & Patterson, E. (1972). Drinking attitudes and behavior of high school students in Kentucky. *Quarterly Journal of Studies on Alcohol, 33*(3), 635-646.

Kaplan, H. B., Martin, S. S., & Robbins, C. (1984). Pathways to adolescent drug use: Self-controls and early substance use. *Journal of Health and Social Behavior, 25,* 270-289.

Kinder, B. N., Pape, N. E., & Walfish, S. (1980). Drug and alcohol education programs: A review of outcome studies. *The International Journal of the Addictions, 15*(7), 1035-1054.

Lange, A. J., & Jakubowski, P. (1976). *Responsible assertive behavior.* Champaign, IL: Research Press.

Lewis, C. E., & Lewis, M. (1984). Peer pressure and risk-taking behaviors in children. *American Journal of Public Health, 74*(6), 580-584.

Lieberman, F., Caroff, P., & Gottesfeld, M. (1973). *Before addiction: How to help youth.* New York: Behavioral Publications.

Linblad, R. A. (1983). *Bulletin on Narcotics, 35*(3), 41-52.

Lowman, C., Hubbard, R. L., Rachal, J. V., & Cavanaugh, E. R. (1982). Facts for planning: Adolescentr marijuana and alcohol use. *Alcohol Health and Research World, 6*(3), 69-75.

MacKay, J. R. (1961). Clinical observation on adolescent problem drinkers. *Quarterly Journal of Studies on Alcohol, 22,* 124-134.

Mayer, J. E., & Filstead, W. J. (1980). Adolescence and alcohol: A theoretical model. In J. Mayer & W. Filstead (Eds.), *Adolescence and alcohol.* Cambridge, MA: Ballinger Publishing Co.

Mayer, W. (1983). Alcohol abuse and alcoholism: The psychologist's role in prevention, research, and treatment. *American Psychologist, 38*(10), 1116-1121.

Montemayor, R. (1982). The relationship between parent-adolescent conflict and the amount of time adolescents spend alone with parents and peers. *Child Development, 53,* 1512-1519.

Moore, M. (1988). *Drug trafficking* (Crime File Study Guide). Washington, DC: U. S. Department of Justice, National Institute of Justice.

National Institute on Drug Abuse. (1985). *National household survey on drugs.* Washington, DC: Author.

National Institute on Drug Abuse. (1987). *Second triennial report to congress on drug abuse and drug abuse research.* Washington, DC: Author

Newcomb, M., Maddahian, E., & Bentler, P. M. (1986). Risk factors for drug use among adolescents: Concurrent and longitudinal analyses. *American Journal of Public Health, 76*(5), 525-531.

Okel, S. (March 15, 1984). Number one killer of youth. *The Georgia Bulletin,* p. 11.

Patterns of drug use. (1987-88, Fall/Winter). *ISR Newsletter,* p. 3, 6.

Patterson, G. R. (1981). *Coercive family processes.* Eugene, OR: Castalia.

Pentz, M. A. (1983). Prevention of adolescent substance abuse through social skill development. In T. Glynn, C. Leukefeld, & J. Ludford (Eds.), *Preventing adolescent drug abuse: Intervention strategies* (NIDA Research Monograph 47). Rockville, MD: DHHS.

Petersen, A. C., & Hamburg, B. A. (1986). Adolescence: A developmental approach to problems and psychopathology. *Behavior Therapy, 17*(5), 480-499.

Pittman, D. J., & Snyder, C. R. (Eds.). (1962). *Society, culture and drinking patterns.* Carbondale: Southern Illinois University Press.

Prendergast, T. J., & Schafer, E. F. (1984). Correlates of drinking and drunkenness among high school students. *Quarterly Journal of Studies on Alcohol, 35,* 232-242.

Pulkkinen, L. (1983). Youthful smoking and drinking in a longitudinal perspective. *Journal of Youth and Adolescence, 12,* 253-283.

Rees, C. D., & Wilborn, B. L. (1983). Correlates of drug abuse in adolescents: A comparison of families of drug users with families of non-drug users. *Journal of Youth and Adolescence, 12,* 55-63.

Robin, A. L. (1981). A controlled evaluation of problem-solving communication training with parent-adolescent conflict. *Behavior Therapy, 12,* 593-609.

Robin, A. L., & Foster, S. L. (1984). Problem-solving communication training: A behavioral family systems approach to parent-adolescent conflict. In P. Karoly & J. Steffen (Eds.), *Adolescent behavior disorders: Foundations and contemporary concerns.* Lexington, MA: D. C. Heath.

Robin, A. L., Kent, R., O'Leary, K. D., Foster, S., & Prinz, R. (1977). An approach to teaching parents and adolescents problem-solving communication skills: A preliminary report. *Behavior Therapy, 8,* 639-643.

Schinke, S. P., & Gilchrist, L. D. (1984). *Life skills counseling with adolescents.* Baltimore: University Park Press.

Schinke, S. P., & Gilchrist, L. D. (1985). Preventing substance abuse with children and adolescents. *Journal of Consulting and Clinical Psychology, 53*(5), 596-602.

Smith, K. A., & Forehand, R. (in press). Parent-adolescent conflict: Comparison and prediction of the perceptions of mothers, fathers, and daughters in a non-clinic sample. *Journal of Early Adolescence.*

Sutherland, E., & Cressey, D. (1970). *Criminology.* Philadelphia: J. B. Lippincott Co.

Swisher, J. D. (1976). An educational policy for school prevention: Rationale and research. *Contemporary Policy Issues, 4,* 27-35.

Taking drugs on the job. (1983, August 22). *Newsweek,* pp. 52-60.

Turanski, J. J. (1983). Researching and treating youth with alcohol related problems: A comprehensive approach. *Alcohol Health and Research World, 7*(4), 3-9.

U. S. Jaycees. (1983). *Drinking myths.* Madison: Wisconsin Clearinghouse.

U. S. National Institute on Drug Abuse. (1982). *Statistical abstract of the U. S. national data book and guide to sources* (103rd ed.) (pp. 123, Tables 195 and 196). Washington, DC: U. S. Department of Commerce, Bureau of the Census.

West, L. J., Maxwell, D. S., Noble, E. P., & Solomon, D. H. (1984). Alcoholism. *Annals of Internal Medicine, 100*(3), 405-416.

Williams, R. L., & long, J. D. (1979). *Toward a self-managed lifestyle.* Boston: Houghton Mifflin Co.

Wodarski, J. S. (1981). *Role of research in clinical practice.* Baltimore: University Park Press.

Wodarski, J. S. (1987a). Evaluating a social learning approach to teaching adolescents about alcohol and driving: A multiple variable evaluation. *Journal of Social Service Research, 10*(2/2/4), 121-144.

Wodarski, J. S. (1987b). A social learning approach to teaching adolescents about drinking and driving: A multiple variable follow-up evaluation. *Journal of Behavior Therapy and Experimental PLsiychiatry, 18*(a), 51-60.

Wodarski, J. S. (1987c). Teaching adolescents about alcohol and driving: A two-year follow-up. *Journal of Drug Education, 17*(4), 327-344.

Wodarski, J. S. (1988). Teaching adolescents about alcohol and driving. *Journal of Alcohol and Drug Education, 33*(3), 46-57.

Wodarski, J. S., & Fisher, A. P. (1986). The alteration of adolescent DUI: A macro approach. *Alcoholism Treatment Quarterly, 3*(2), 153-162.

Wodarski, J. S., & Hoffman, S. D. (1984). Alcohol education for adolescents. *Social Work in Education, 6*(2), 69-92.

Wodarski, L. A., Adelson, C., Tidball, M., & Wodarski, J. S. (1980). Teaching nutrition by teams-games-tournaments. *Journal of Nutrition Education, 12*(2), 61-65.

Chapter 6

ADOLESCENT SUICIDE:
A REVIEW OF INFLUENCES AND THE MEANS
FOR PREVENTION

John S. Wodarski and Pamela Harris

CONSIDERABLE EFFORT has been made during the past decade to assimilate information and to elucidate causes of adolescent suicide—one of the most difficult problems facing America today. Traditionally, adolescence has been viewed as a carefree period of life. In reality, however, the transition from childhood to adulthood is fraught with psychological, sociological, and physical changes (Elkind, 1984a, 1984b).

The epidemic of adolescent suicide closely resembles French sociologist Emile Durkheim's (1951) definition of **anomic suicide,** which arises from a rapid change in the social order or social norms. Roberts (1975) writes of anomic suicide: "The individual becomes uncertain of the appropriate behavior expected of him/her and experiences a state of anomic normlessness, an unbridgeable gap between aspirations and achievements where individual passions are out of control" (p. 27).

Growing up today is different from growing up in the 1960s. Then, most children had relatively warm, caring families; stable school environments; and trusting adults. In contrast, a significant percentage of today's teenagers are maturing in a state of relative fear. Many adolescents are experiencing family breakups or are observing them in their friends' homes (Wodarski, 1982; Wattenberg, 1986). Demographic trends have led to overcrowded schools in which an impersonal atmosphere creates a sense of alienation among the students (Holinger & Offer, 1981; Packard, 1983; Wenz, 1979).

The focus of the literature, however, is on the inability of children and teenagers to form close relationships with adults at home and outside the family structure. The alienation experienced by children and adolescents has long-term effects on the individual's outlook on moral and social issues. Alienation breeds a lack of trust within the child (Arnold et al., 1983; Coles, 1983). Society in the 1980s tends to ally children with children and adults with adults in social settings. Because of this lack of intergenerational interaction, adolescents feel rejected (Kaplan, Robbins, & Martin, 1983).

The suicidal adolescent envisions an environment of helplessness and hopelessness (Berkovitz, 1981; Miller, 1981; Petzel & Riddle, 1981; Tabachnick, 1981). Davis (1983) noted that suicidal adolescents, when placed in highly intensive emotional situations (for example, the breakup of a relationship or conflict with parents), suffer from a helpless feeling of "tunnel vision" in which they fail to see options. This constricted view affords the teenager the opportunity to deal only with difficulties in the present frame of reference (U. S. Congress, 1984a). Topol and Reznikoff (1982) have suggested that external locus of control by the teenager contributes to this sense of hopelessness.

No theoretical formulation that can adequately account for the prediction of suicide is supported by data. Thus, in this chapter, current research on adolescent suicide is examined using the following conceptual foci: depression, stress, family, and peers. Background information on statistical trends is highlighted, and causal factors and practice considerations to help adolescents are discussed.

STATISTICAL TRENDS IN ADOLESCENT SUICIDE

After accidents and homicides, suicide is the leading cause of death in the 15- to 24-year-old age group (U. S. Vital Statistics, 1978). The adolescent population is at greatest risk of committing suicide, and the risk is increasing (Frederick, 1978; Toolan, 1975). Between 1960 and 1980, the suicide rate rose from 5.2 to 12.3 per 100,000 for this age group, marking a 136 percent increase. The rate is increasing most rapidly for white males (U. S. Congress, 1984a).

Methodological flaws in the classification of cause of death confound suicide data reporting. Because of the difficulty in obtaining unbiased material, the accuracy of reported cases is questionable. For situations in which accidents are probable suicides, the cause may not be listed as such, either because of a lack of investigative staff or because of parental pressure for confidentiality (Mishara, 1975; Pokorny, 1975). In many cases, suicide may be the actual cause of deaths that are reported formally as homicides.

Deaths by suicide that actually are reported appear to reflect only part of the problem. Studies in which the extent of attempted and completed suicides was examined have shown that for every contemplated suicide, there are an estimated 50 to 150 attempts (McIntire et al., 1977). Studies on teenage suicide attempts and death have found previous suicidal behavior in 40 to 50 percent of the cases (Gibbs, 1981; Shaffer & Fisher, 1981). Attempts at suicide appear to be cries for help in dealing with a problem that the teenager perceives as insurmountable (Smith, 1981; U. S. Congress, 1984a).

Girls attempt suicide more often than boys (Korrella, 1972; Miller, Chiles, & Barnes, 1982). Boys, however, are more successful in completing the act, because they use more potent, foolproof methods (Davis, 1983; Garfinkel, Froese, & Hood, 1982; Hawton, 1982; Rosenthal, 1981). Boys frequently use guns, ropes, or automobiles. Girls often fear disfigurement and therefore use less lethal methods, such as pills or wrist slashing.

Self-imposed risks and self-destructive behavior (antecedents of suicidal behavior in reported homicides) frequently are observed (Farberow, 1980; Holinger, 1979; Klagsbrun, 1981). Self-destructive behavior and marginally intentional suicidal behavior include situations such as repetitive driving-under-the-influence offenses, frequent drug and marijuana use, and accident proneness because of the individual's neglect of safety (Marohn et al., 1982; Miller, 1981; Nielsen, 1983; Sartore, 1976).

DYNAMICS OF ADOLESCENCE RELEVANT TO SUICIDE

Adolescence is a period of intense change. Sexual maturity, with heterosexual and homosexual impulses, develops at the same time as the need for separation from parents and individuation becomes more pronounced (Berkovitz, 1981; Blos, 1979; Bratter, 1975; Getz et al., 1983). Miller (1981) defines adolescence as a process that is valuable in the development of autonomy. The teenager experiences a new consciousness of self and has the need to reevaluate values (Konopka, 1983). Values clarification becomes of primary importance and the teenage years become a testing ground for future growth (Arnold et al., 1983; DenHouter, 1981).

Physical, psychological, and social developmental changes unique to adolescence make this an especially stressful period. Bloom (1980) views cognitive development and an environment in which the teenager receives realistic feedback as crucial to the separation process. According to one view, suicide attempts reflect a breakdown in adolescent reality testing (Crumley, 1982).

Although affiliation needs are great during adolescence, the ability to become autonomous and self-sufficient must be developed. However, loneliness, for many teenagers, accompanies these feelings (Tabachnick, 1981).

During the individuation process, the ability to cope with changing life situations and growth in self-esteem are pursued. O'Malley and Bachman (1983) found significant increases in self-esteem from age 13 to early adulthood. A deficit in this process has far-reaching implications for the individual. Chronic inability to cope ranks high as a predictor in suicide attempts (Crumley, 1982; Greuling & DeBlassie, 1980; Jacobs & Teicher, 1967; Linehan et al., 1983). A distorted self-image or lack of self-esteem deeply affects the teenager in future endeavors in his/her environment. These problems, in turn, generate the rejection so often exhibited in suicidal behavior (Glaser, 1978; Rosenkrantz, 1978). Walch (1977) analyzed the differences between male and female attempters and found that male attempters had a severe sense of disesteem, whereas female attempters experienced aberrations from external sources (such as school or peers). At this developmental stage, when growth is frustrated and anger is repressed, suicide becomes a reality (Berkovitz, 1981).

In situations in which identity problems are present, teenagers may be overly dependent on family relationships for affirmation of their identities, while family members may discourage separations (Harbin, 1977; Heillig, 1980; Pfeffer, 1981). Consequently, the teenager may become compulsive in interpersonal relations. The adolescent suicide attempt in these cases has been conceptualized as an impulsive act intended to resolve the conflicted situation (Rosenkrantz, 1978).

CAUSAL FACTORS IN ADOLESCENT SUICIDE

Suicidal behavior is the result of the teenager's dysfunctional adjustment to psychological and environmental circumstances. Aspects of depression and stress have been cited in research studies as prodromal clues in attempted and completed suicides (Davis, 1983). The roles of family and peers have been examined in the same contexts.

Depression

Adolescents naturally experience depression as part of the maturation process; however, the intensity and severity of depression is a factor in the adolescent's psychological health (Nichtern, 1982). The emotional states of suicidal individuals are indecisive — the wish to live versus the wish to die plays at their emotions. Research by Kovacs and Beck (1977) on those who attempt suicide found this internal debate in more than 50 percent of the participants tested, using a Wish-to-Live/Wish-to-Die Scale.

Intense depression has been found to be the most prevalent characteristic of suicidal youths (Calhoun, 1972; Friedman et al., 1984; Gibbs, 1981; Marks & Haller, 1977; Miller, 1975; Tishler & McKenry, 1983). Vegetative symptoms of depression include the following: mood variations, sleep disturbances, fatigue and loss of energy, and appetite changes (Rosenblatt, 1981; Tishler & McKenry, 1982). In the school setting, a decline in academic performance or a withdrawal from peers and extracurricular activities is an indicator of depression (DenHouter, 1981; Glaser, 1967; Greuling & DeBlassie, 1980; Petzel & Riddle, 1981).

Loner adolescents (who present themselves as having no significant friendships during the critical years) are especially vulnerable to depression and suicidal ideation. Miller (1981) and Hawton (1982) found a number of adolescents were depressed for years because of earlier deprivation or a profound sense of emptiness in their lives (Hawton, 1982). Individuals who attempt suicide are characterized by a high degree of alienation from peer group interactions (Madison, 1978).

Alcohol and drug abuse are defense mechanisms used to combat depression. Excessive alcohol ingestion may lead to loss of control over suicidal impulses (Greuling & DeBlassie, 1980). Greuling and DeBlassie (1980) studied statistics from several large cities and found that more than 50 percent of teenagers who had committed suicide had a history of moderate to severe drinking and drug abuse. Researchers have noted that acting-out behaviors and discipline problems exhibited by adolescents many times mask depression (Greuling & DeBlassie, 1980;

Nielsen, 1983). Suicide attempts by adolescents have been viewed as a means of dealing with depression and regaining control over their lives (Getz et al., 1983).

Depression concerns mental health professionals because it has increased sharply within the past decade. In citing Kohut's (1971, 1980) studies of troubled teenagers, Lewis (1982) noted that teenagers experienced chronic bouts of depression and projected themselves as being overwhelmed easily and having a sense of being enraged.

In one study, the Beck Depression Inventory and six adjustment items were administered to a group of 63 seventh and eighth graders to determine the occurrence of depression (Albert & Beck, 1975). Thirty-three percent of those students were experiencing moderate to severe depression, and 35 percent acknowledged current suicidal ideation. Difficulties in school and social adjustment and the measured severity of the depression showed a high correlation.

Stress

The debilitating physical and psychological effects of stress on the human body have been studied in depth. Compared with other cultures, Americans traditionally place themselves under great stress because of their extremely high expectations. This practice has filtered down gradually to increase the expectations that parents place on children. Research shows that this emphasis on achievement contributes to the current suicidal crisis (McAraney, 1979; U. S. Congress, 1984b).

Testing and grading procedures in American school systems tend to label children at an early age according to the failure-success model. A correlation between school failure and suicide has been noted (Davis, 1983). School failure significantly contributes to the stressful, helpless feelings demonstrated by teenagers who have a history of making poor grades (Sartore, 1976). White males particularly are susceptible to performance pressures (Holinger & Offer, 1981). In Japan, the high suicide rate among male and female adolescents has been linked to stress created by the school examination system in which adolescents compete for the coveted selection into college (Farber, 1968; World Health Organization, 1975).

Stress is especially great for U. S. teenagers whose parents live vicariously through their children's achievements (Madison, 1978). Overachievers as well as underachievers are at a distinct risk for suicide. Research showed that the unusually high expectations of overachievers led to an unhealthy mental attitude, whereas a sense of futility burdened those adolescents who were labeled learning disabled (U. S. Congress, 1984b). After a three-year study of adolescents who attempted suicide, Kenny (1979) proposed that an unrecognized learning disability may be a factor in a considerable percentage of adolescent suicide attempts.

Stress also can be a factor in situations in which an adolescent's internal and external conflicts have not been resolved, such as inadequate separation from a parent (Nielsen, 1983). Many disturbed adolescents see suicide as a form of conflict resolution (Miller, 1980).

Stress was a distinctive feature of completed suicides according to Sanborn, Sanborn, and Cimbolic (1973), who investigated completed teenage suicides within a two-year period in New Hampshire. By conducting "psychological autopsies" on each individual, the researchers concluded that acute stress was present in the lives of more than 50 percent of subjects studied before their deaths.

Drastic changes in a teenager's life (such as death of parent, firing from a job, rejection by a team or school) also precipitate stress. Significant others, who likely are aware of these events, should be alert to their impact on the teenager's life and be able to recognize certain behaviors as attempts to adjust to the particular circumstances (McBrien, 1983).

Family Influences

The family as the integral formation model has a distinct effect on the child. In the early years, foundations of trust and love are established for the child within the home. The individual's ability to function is determined largely by his or her psychological growth during this period.

The American family has been in a state of flux for the past 20 years. The growing incidence of family dissolutions, and the resulting single-parent households along with the attendant life-style, makes childhood a difficult period. To accommodate new parenting situations, old patterns of child rearing are being put aside. Sociological researchers tend to view the phenomenon of adolescent suicide as a reflection of this turmoil in American families (Hawton, 1982; Petzel & Riddle, 1981; Swenson & Rabin, 1981). Hendin (1975) has suggested that there is a trend toward devaluation of family and children and an atmosphere that lacks intimacy and affection. Experiences in environments that are non-supportive and overly hostile contribute to the development of suicidal personality characteristics.

Studies of suicide attempts by hospitalized patients and of completed suicides within a school year have demonstrated that family disruptions and disintegration played a significant role in the maladaptation of these individuals (U. S. Congress, 1984b). Close to one-half (43%) of cases reviewed by Litt, Cuskey, and Rudd (1983) reported that a family argument preceded a suicide attempt. A family environment where the possibility of divorce or separation was discussed openly was found to be troubling for teenagers and a factor in suicide attempts.

Jacobs and Teicher (1967) and Anderson (1981) have indicated the importance of the family in the adolescent's functioning. By using life history charts, much information can be ascertained about the adolescent's family. The life history chart usually substantiates the theory that a progression of unhappy life events rather than one traumatic event precipitates the suicidal act. A history of psychiatric illness and previous suicides characterize many of these families (Friedman et al., 1984). Other studies have attributed this background to patterns of inadequate role modeling throughout generations (Holinger & Offer, 1982; Ray & Johnson, 1983; Tishler, 1982; Tishler & McKenry, 1982). A parent's chronic illness (lasting more than 24 weeks) also has been shown to be a factor in adolescent depression and suicidal ideation (Friedman et al., 1984; Murphy & Wetzel, 1982).

In a discussion of the influence of family on suicide, the emotional and physical ties of adolescents with their parents must be considered. McKenry, Tishler, and Kelly (1982) compared 46 "attempters" with a comparable number of "non-attempters" from an emergency room population. To evaluate level of depression, family conflict, and family cohesion, the subjects were administered a battery of tests. The results revealed the attempters' negative perception of their relationships with their parents. The attempters also felt that their mothers were less interested in them than did the non-attempters. Attempters' fathers, in comparison with parents of non-attempters, had low self-esteem, and attempters' mothers reported suicidal ideation. Moreover, alcohol use was more prevalent in attempters' mothers and fathers, a distinguishing trait also noted by Garfinkel, Froese, and Hood (1982) and McIntire et al. (1977). Positive traits discerned in non-attempters' families included healthy identity formation, prosocial ego development, and a sense of intimacy.

A lack of communication within the family has been explored as a variable in attempted and completed suicides (Abraham, 1978). Sanborn et al. (1973) viewed family difficulties in communicating as a primary problem, and Abraham (1978) noted the families' restrictions in responding to other family members' needs and in self-disclosure. Housman (1981) noted that a lack of empathic communication between mother and daughter can lead to suicidal ideation.

In studies by Uber (1983) and Harbin (1977), a high degree of hostility was expressed by attempters toward their parents but was accompanied by a sense of guilt on the part of the teenagers. These behaviors resulted from the teenager's difficulty in separating from parents while at the same time developing a sense of autonomy.

Several investigators have examined the link between childhood loss and later attempted suicide. A childhood that is characterized by parental discord and by frequent intentional parental separations from the child was shown to be associated with later suicide attempts, although parental loss because of death was not shown to precipitate suicidal intentions (Crook & Raskin, 1975; Nielsen, 1983). Parental deprivation and rejection can lead to what Dorpat (1975) has called a **rejection hypothesis**, in which the teenager internalizes rejection and it later becomes a factor in adolescent suicide attempts.

Peer Involvement

When teenagers attempt to form separate identities from their parents, they commence earnest involvement with peers. At school, adolescents begin to ascertain their strengths and limitations academically and socially. Adolescents' ability to handle the rigors of this adjustment period depends predominately on their previous experiences. Sexual identification and the addition of a significant other create a push-pull effect, in which the teenager is pushed into adulthood while still desiring the security of childhood. Tabachnick (1981) has focused on the adolescent's fear that he or she "cannot make it."

The ability of adolescents to interact with peers significantly influences their later social adjustment. Janes et al. (1979) studied boys in late childhood and early adolescence and again 12 years later. The researchers concluded that failure to get along with peers during childhood and adolescence is associated closely with a spectrum of dysfunctional adult behaviors.

In the search for the components of their personality, teenagers scrutinize those around them and determine their own self-worth. When troubled youths view themselves as surrounded by well-functioning peers, their self-esteem is lowered and they may contemplate suicide (Holinger & Offer, 1981).

When youths are desolate, they will seek the assistance of peers to discuss their feelings. Survey studies have validated the idea that teenagers, when experiencing suicidal thoughts, invariably will select a friend over other choices such as a relative, teacher, or nurse (Greuling & De-Blassie, 1980; Ross, 1980). Thus, peer involvement should be given the highest priority in a clinical program, because potential suicides emit clear signals that can warn those around attempters of impending danger if those individuals are knowledgeable about such signals and their meanings (Ray & Johnson, 1983).

Social Work Practice Considerations

Acknowledgment of a problem is the first step toward resolution. Substantial research has been devoted to adolescent suicide. Those individuals who work with youths can demonstrate their concern about adolescent suicide by developing prevention programs aimed at three groups: (1) adolescents, (2) parents, and (3) school teachers and counselors. The subject matter should include a discussion with the teenager of suicide prevention techniques and the adaptive skills necessary to cope with the stresses of life. Many teenagers struggle to accept the give and take of everyday living. Because research has indicated that suicidal ideation occurs during latency childhood, introducing a suicide prevention program at the middle-school level would be appropriate (Pfeffer, 1981). Programs may be incorporated into health education courses or worked into a discussion group at youth groups associated with churches and community agencies (Tishler & Jacobs, 1983).

Many short courses on improving communication skills are available to organizations; such courses could be adapted for classroom use. Not only would a communication skills course be helpful to teenagers as they interact with their peers, but the course also would be a great asset to adolescents when they are outside of the school environment.

Parents should be introduced to the idea of suicide prevention. Parent-teacher association meetings provide an excellent forum for discussing the problem. The program's main thrust should be heightening communication skills between child and parent, because lack of communication consistently has been shown to have an effect on suicidal ideation. Focusing on the causes and signals of suicide should be part of the program for the parents, and teachers and school personnel should be trained to spot potential suicides ("Preventing Teenage Suicide," 1983).

Teachers need to be acutely aware of the clues of suicidal behavior. Gordon (1979) found that secondary school teachers have little knowledge concerning adolescent suicide. However, the teachers have expressed positive attitudes toward learning about teacher intervention in dealing with this crisis. The time the adolescent spends in school and the ability to view the troubled adolescent outside the confines of the home affords school professionals an opportunity to assess the potential for suicide and to make appropriate referrals (Grob, Klein, & Eisen, 1983; Smith, 1976).

Charlotte Ross (1980) spearheaded a successful suicide prevention project in the school system of San Mateo, California. Students and teachers were introduced to the basic information about suicidal behavior. School personnel were enlightened about presuicidal behavior and ways that they could respond effectively. In her interviews with teachers about suicide prevention, Ross found that individuals are cautious when speaking of suicides. Many feel that a discussion of the subject can be suggestive and negative for teenagers. Contrary to this notion, Ross reiterates that talking about suicidal feelings with school personnel can be extremely helpful to suicidal adolescents and can help them ventilate emotions.

Parents and professionals can make diligent efforts to develop active listening skills. Through such listening skills, they may be able to discern indirect clues regarded as whispers for help. Loaded statements such as "My life is empty" or "I have these weird thoughts" should alert anyone who is close to a teenager to the possibility of suicide (McBrien, 1983).

PRACTICE PARADIGM

A surprising fact about suicide prevention is that adolescents want to learn about suicide prevention. Between 80 and 90 percent of approximately 25,000 high school students surveyed during the course of several studies wanted to learn the facts about suicide prevention (Carlson, 1981; Elkind, 1984a, 1984b; Smith, 1976).

Often, the obstacle to useful, comprehensive prevention education is teachers' discomfort in dealing with the dynamics of suicide. Teachers may lack well-organized and easy-to-understand delivery methods for educating youths about suicide. In contrast, when educational packets on other topics of interest to adolescents, such as substance abuse, have been developed and presented to teachers, and the teachers have been trained to use the material, the teachers have been more receptive and eager to use prevention in their curriculum (Wodarski, 1987).

Effective, comprehensive methods of teaching youths about suicide prevention are imperative. To be effective with youths, preventive efforts should be made during the most receptive time, which seems to be the early adolescent years, following the influence of the parental-home setting and coinciding with the rise in peer influence. This phase usually begins at age 12 or 13 years, most often in the seventh and eighth grades. Based on the facts reviewed, the authors have tested a practice paradigm for suicide prevention that includes the following components: cognitive self-management of depression, problem solving, family interaction skills development, and peer skills development.

Cognitive Self-Management of Depression

There appear to be continuities between childhood and adult depression. Depressed children apparently are capable of evoking negative expectations about the future and share certain cognitive attributes of depressed adults. Hopelessness, depression, and suicidal intent also appear to be related for children and adults. Data indicate that cognitive approaches to altering adult cognitions may be appropriate for adolescents. Thus, the intervention is an attempt to alter what the adolescent thinks to change behavior. The aim is to reduce the frequency of cognitions that elicit undesirable behaviors (Hulbert & Sipprelle, 1978). Therefore, the focus of this intervention is on the cognitive self-statements that the adolescent makes. Depressive self-statements are thought to result from a faulty belief system and thinking pattern (Meichenbaum, 1975).

Cognitive theorists believe there are four types of cognitive distortions. The curriculum includes means to alter all four of the distortions.

(1) **Arbitrary inference** is the process of drawing a conclusion when evidence is lacking or is contrary to the conclusion.

(2) **Overgeneralization** is the process of making an unjustified generalization on the basis of a single incident.

(3) **Magnification** is the propensity to exaggerate the meaning or significance of a particular event.

(4) **Cognitive deficiency** is the disregard of an important aspect of a life situation; adolescents with this cognitive distortion ignore, fail to integrate, or do not use information derived from experience. Consequently, the adolescents behave as though they have a defect in their system of expectations (Beck, 1976).

Theorists have emphasized the cognitive aspects of depression. Beck (1970) assigned a primary position to a cognitive triad consisting of a profoundly negative view of the self, of the outside world, and of the future. This triad is seen as the key to the consequences of depression, such as the lack of motivation, the affective state, and other ideational and behavioral manifestations. The depressed person's cognitions lead to misinterpretations of experiences; hence, many of the secondary responses are logical consequences of such misinterpretations. The depressed person is locked in an insoluble situation of further despair (Calhoun, Adams, & Mitchell, 1974). Therefore, cognitive responses that can be altered include sense of hopelessness, self-condemnation and self-defeating thoughts, low self-esteem, tensions, death wishes, and sense of helplessness.

Problem Solving

Suicidal adolescents have been identified as high risk in coping with the academic and social daily problems of living. Therefore, including problem-solving techniques is an important component of the curriculum. The problem-solving approach involves, among other skills, generating information and solutions, choosing and implementing strategies by understanding the consequences, using consequences to modify a behavior, and confirming the outcome (Robin & Foster, 1984; Wodarski & Hedrick, 1987).

Family Interaction Skills

In the family intervention component, parents participate in a four-week program conducted by social workers in which they meet in groups for two hours each week. The dynamics of suicide prevention are covered in the written materials distributed and in the first two-hour group session.

Sessions two and three teach problem-solving and communication skills for conflict resolution based on Robin and Foster's (1984) work. The five steps of problem solving are delineated as follows: (1) problem definition, (2) generation of alternate solutions, (3) decision making, (4) planning solution implementation, and (5) renegotiation. Initially, parents are presented the steps in a formal manner. Parents then discuss the steps in the group and role play how to use the procedures. During the role play, group members attempt to solve problems of adolescents of other group members.

Information also is presented on the use of positive and negative control with adolescents, with a focus on increasing the use of positive reinforcement for appropriate behavior rather than coercive processes such as negative reinforcement and punishment (Forehand & McMahon, 1981; Patterson, 1981).

In the final session, problem-solving techniques, communication training and positive reinforcement procedures are integrated and applied to suicide prevention. The social workers conducting the program emphasize that using communication and problem-solving skills and positive reinforcement will result in a better relationship with adolescents (specifically, better communication and less conflict) and, therefore, reduce the probability of suicide.

Peer Skills

Improving participants' interpersonal skills and altering their negative self-perceptions are components or goals of suicide prevention. These goals can be accomplished by focusing on adolescent peer interaction.

Lange and Jakubowski (1976) as cited in Wodarski and Hedrick (1987) have developed methods to use for teaching the participants how to interact with others in meaningful and satisfying ways. Important interactional skills include how to introduce one's self, how to initiate and continue conversations, and how to give and receive compliments.

SUMMARY

The solution to adolescent suicide requires maximum effort by societal forces capable of effecting change. Families, schools, peers, communities, businesses, and the media all possess influence to eradicate this social problem. The campaign cannot be waged from only one front. Combined cooperative efforts are essential. The responsibility must be shared for previous actions that have perpetuated the problem and for working toward mutual goals and solutions.

Students, teachers, and parents have expressed need and interest in receiving training and education in suicide prevention. Yet, despite the widespread concern over the physical, social, and emotional aspects of adolescence, there have been few scientifically evaluated preventive programs. This practice paradigm represents a new concept in suicide prevention. The intervention is a unique combination of presentation of educational material in a manner that encourages peer support, use of a group reward structure and participatory learning, and family involvement.

Chapter 6 has addressed the third leading cause of death among youths — adolescent suicide. Depression, stress, family, and peer factors that impinge on adolescents and predispose them to suicide were reviewed. The role of professionals in prevention efforts was examined and a practice paradigm for identifying and helping suicidal adolescents was outlined.

REFERENCES

Abraham, Y. (1978). Patterns of communication and rejection in families of suicidal adolescents. *Dissertation Abstracts International, 38*(Sec. A), 4669.

Albert, N., & Beck, A. T. (1975). Incidences of depression in early adolescence: A preliminary study. *Journal of Youth and Adolescence, 4,* 301-307.

Anderson, D. R. (1981). Diagnosis and prediction of suicidal risk among adolescents. In C. Wells & I. Stuart (Eds.), *Self destructive behavior in children and adolescents.* New York: Van Nostrand Reinhold.

Arnold, L. E. et al. (1983). Unprevented alienation: Case illustration and group discussion. In L. Arnold et al (Eds.), *Preventing adolescent alienation.* Lexington, MA: D. C. Heath & Co.

Beck, A. (1970). Cognitive therapy: Nature and relation to behavior therapy. *Behavior Therapy, 1,* 184-200.

Beck, A. (1976). *Cognitive therapy and the emotional disorders.* New York: International Universities Press.

Berkovitz, I. H. (1981). Feelings of powerlessness and the role of violent actions in adolescents. In S. Feinstein et al. (Eds.), *Adolescent psychiatry: Developmental and clinical studies* (Vol. 9). Chicago: University of Chicago Press.

Bloom, M. (1980). *Adolescent parental separation.* New York: Gardner Press.

Blos, P. (1979). *The adolescent passage.* New York: International Universities Press.

Bratter, T. E. (1975). Responsible therapeutic eros: The psychotherapist who cares enough to define and enforce behavior limits with potential suicidal adolescents. *Counseling Psychologist, 5,* 97-104.

Calhoun, J. F. (1972). *Abnormal psychology.* New York: Random House.

Calhoun, K. S., Adams, H. E., & Mitchell, K. M. (1974). *Innovative treatment methods in psychopathology.* New York: Wiley.

Carlson, G. A. (1981). The phenomenology of adolescent depression. In S. Feinstein et al. (Eds.), *Adolescent psychiatry: Developmental and clinical studies* (Vol. 9). Chicago: University of Chicago Press.

Coles, R. (1983). Alienated youth and humility for the professions. In L. Arnold (Ed.), *Preventing adolescent alienation.* Lexington, MA: D. C. Heath & Co.

Crook, T., & Raskin, A. (1975). Association of childhood parental loss with attempted suicide and depression. *Journal of Consulting and Clinical Psychology, 43,* 277.

Crumley, F. E. (1982). The adolescent suicide attempt: A cardinal symptom of a serious psychiatric disorder. *American Journal of Psychotherapy, 36,* 158-165.

Davis, P. A. (1983). *Suicidal adolescents.* Springfield, IL: Charles C Thomas.

DenHouter, K. V. (1981). To silence one's self: A brief analysis of the literature on adolescent suicide. *Child Welfare, 60,* 2-10.

Dorpat, T. (1975). Dyscontrol and suicidal behavior. In A. Roberts (Ed.), *Self-destructive behavior.* Springfield, IL: Charles C Thomas.

Durkheim, E. (1951). *Suicide: A study in sociology.* New York: Free Press.

Elkind, D. (1984a). *All grown up and no place to go.* Reading, MA: Addison-Wesley.

Elkind, D. (1984b). *The hurried child.* Reading, MA: Addison-Wesley.

Farber, M. L. (1968). *Theories of suicide.* New York: Funk & Wagnalls.

Farberow, N. (1980). *The many faces of suicide: Indirect self-destructive behavior.* New York: McGraw-Hill

Forehand, R., & McMahon, R. J. (1981). *Helping the non-compliant child: A clinician's guide to parent training.* New York: Guilford Press.

Frederick, C. J. (1978). Current trends in suicidal behavior in the United States. *American Journal of Psychotherapy, 32,* 172-200.

Friedman, R. C. et al. (1984). Family history of illness in the seriously suicidal adolescent: A life cycle approach. *American Journal of Orthopsychiatry, 54,* 390-397.

Garfinkel, B. D., Froese, A., & Hood, J. (1982). Suicide attempts in children and adolescents. *American Journal of Psychiatry, 139,* 1257-1261.

Getz, W. L. et al. (1983). *Brief counseling with suicidal persons.* Lexington, MA: D. C. Heath & Co.

Gibbs, J. T. (1981). Depression and suicidal behavior among delinquent females. *Journal of Youth and Adolescence, 10,* 159-167.

Glaser, K. (1967). Masked depression in children and adolescents. *American Journal of Psychotherapy, 21,* 565-574.

Glaser, K. (1978). The treatment of depressed and suicidal adolescents. *American Journal of Psychotherapy, 32,* 252-269.

Gordon, S. L. (1979). An analysis of the knowledge and attitudes of secondary school teachers concerning suicide among adolescents and intervention in adolescent suicide. *Dissertation Abstracts International, 40*(Sec. A)., 1393-1394.

Greuling, J., & DeBlassie, R. R. (1980). Adolescent suicide. *Adolescence, 15,* 589-601.

Grob, M. C., Klein, A. A., & Eisen, S. V. (1983). The role of the high school professional in identifying suicidal behavior. *Journal of Youth and Adolescence, 12,* 163-173.

Harbin, H. T. (1977). Episodic dyscontrol and family dynamics. *American Journal of Psychiatry, 134,* 1113-1116.

Hawton, K. (1982). Attempted suicide in children and adolescents. *Journal of Child Psychology and Psychiatry and Allied Disciplines, 23,* 497-503.

Heillig, R. J. (1980). Adolescent suicidal behavior: A family system perspective. *Dissertation Abstracts International, 40*(Sec. B), 5813.

Hendin, H. (1975). Growing up dead: Student suicide. *American Journal of Psychotherapy, 29,* 327-338.

Holinger, P. C. (1979). Violent deaths among the young: Recent trends in suicide, homicide, and accidents. *American Journal of Psychiatry, 136*(9), 1144-1147.

Holinger, P. C., & Offer, D. (1981). Perspectives on suicide in adolescence. *Research in Community & Mental Health, 2,* 139-157.

Holinger, P. C., & Offer, D. (1982). Predictions of adolescent suicide: A population model. *American Journal of Psychiatry, 139,* 302-307.

Housman, D. K. (1981). The relationship between suicide behavior in female adolescents and the lack of empathic capacity and differentiation on the part of the mothers. *Dissertation Abstracts International, 42*(Sec. B), 2530.

Hulbert, R. T., & Sipprelle, C. N. (1978). Random sampling of cognitions in alleviating anxiety attacks. *Cognitive Therapy and Research, 2,* 165-169.

Jacobs, J., & Teicher, J. D. (1967). Broken homes and social isolation in attempted suicides of adolescents. *The International Journal of Social Psychiatry, 13,* 139-149.

Janes, C. L. et al. (1979). Problem boys in young adulthood: Teacher's ratings and the twelve year follow-up. *Journal of Youth & Adolescence, 8,* 453-472.

Kaplan, H. B., Robbins, C., & Martin, S. (1983). Antecedents of psychological distress in young adults: Self-rejection, deprivation of social support and life events. *Journal of Health & Social Behavior, 24,* 230-244.

Kenny, T. J. (1979). Visual-motor problems of adolescents who attempt suicide. *Perceptual and Motor Skills, 48,* 599-602.

Klagsbrun, F. (1981). *Too young to die.* New York: Simon & Schuster.

Kohut, H. (1971). *The analysis of the self.* New York: International Universities Press.

Kohut, H. (1980, November). *Self-psychology: Reflections on the present and the future.* Paper presented at the Boston Psychoanalytic Association Symposium on Reflections on Self-Psychology, Boston, MA.

Konopka, G. (1983). Adolescent suicide. *Exceptional Children, 49,* 390-394.

Korrella, K. (1972). Teenage suicidal gestures: A study of suicidal behavior among high school students. *Dissertation Abstracts International, 32*(Sec. A), 5039.

Kovacs, M., & Beck, A. (1977). The wish to die and the wish to live in attempted suicides. *Journal of Clinical Psychology, 33,* 361-365.

Lange, A. J., & Jakubowski, P. (1976). *Responsible assertive behavior.* Champaign, IL: Research Press.

Lewis, M. (1982). Adolescent psychic structure and societal influences. In S. Feinstein et al. (Eds.), *Adolescent psychiatry: Developmental and clinical studies* (Vol. 10). Chicago: University of Chicago Press.

Linehan, M. M. et al. (1983). Reasons for staying alive when you are thinking of killing yourself: The Reason for Living Inventory. *Journal of Consulting and Clinical Psychology, 51,* 276-286.

Litt, I. F., Cuskey, W. R., & Rudd, S. (1983). Emergency room evaluation of the adolescent who attempts suicide: Compliance with follow-up. *Journal of Adolescent Health Care, 4,* 106-108.

Madison, A. (1978). *Suicide and young people.* New York: Seabury Press.

Marks, P. A., & Haller, D. L. (1977). Now I lay me down for keeps: A study of adolescent suicide attempts. *Journal of Clinical Psychology, 33,* 390-400.

Marohn, R. C. et al. (1982). Juvenile delinquents and violent death. In S. Feinstein et al. (Eds.), *Adolescent psychiatry: Developmental and clinical studies* (Vol. 10). Chicago: University of Chicago Press.

McAraney, E. R. (1979). Adolescent and young adult suicide in the United States: A reflection of societal unrest? *Adolescence, 14,* 765-774.

McBrien, R. J. (1983). Are you thinking of killing yourself? Confronting students' suicidal thoughts. *School Counselor, 31,* 75-82.

McIntire, M. et al. (1977). Recurrent adolescent suicidal behavior. *Pediatrics, 60,* 605-608.

McKenry, P., Tishler, C., & Kelley, C. (1982). Adolescent suicide: A comparison of attempters and nonattempters in an emergency room population. *Clinical Pediatrics, 21,* 266-270.

Meichenbaum, D. (1975). Self-instructional methods. In F. Kanfer & A. Goldstein (Eds.), *Helping people change.* New York: Pergamon.

Miller, D. (1980). Treatment of the severely disturbed adolescent. In S. Feinstein et al (Eds.), *Adolescent psychiatry: Developmental and clinical studies* (Vol. 8). Chicago: University of Chicago Press.

Miller, D. (1981). Adolescent suicide: Etiology and treatment. In S. Feinstein et al. (Eds.), *Adolescent psychiatry: Developmental and clinical studies* (Vol. 9). Chicago: University of Chicago Press.

Miller, J. P. (1975). Suicide and adolescence. *Adolescence, 10,* 11-24.

Miller, M. L., Chiles, J. A., & Barnes, V. (1982). Suicide attempters within a delinquent population. *Journal of Consulting & Clinical Psychology, 50,* 491-498.

Mishara, B. L. (1975). The extent of adolescent suicidality. *Psychiatric Opinion, 12,* 32-37.

Murphy, G. E., & Wetzel, R. D. (1982). Family history of suicidal behavior among suicide attempters. *The Journal of Nervous & Mental Disease, 170,* 86-90.

Nichtern, S. (1982). The sociocultural and psychodynamic aspects of the acting-out and violent adolescent. In S. Feinstein et al. (Eds.), *Adolescent psychiatry: Developmental and clinical studies* (Vol. 10). Chicago: University of Chicago Press.

Nielsen, G. (1983). *Borderline and acting out adolescents.* New York: Human Sciences Press.

O'Malley, P. M., & Bachman, J. F. (1983). Self-esteem: Change and stability between ages 13 and 23. *Developmental Psychology, 19,* 257-268.

Packard, V. (1983). *Our endangered children: Growing up in a changing world.* Boston: Little, Brown & Co.

Patterson, G. R. (1981). *Coercive family process.* Eugene, OR: Castalia.

Petzel, S., & Riddle, M. (1981). Adolescent suicide: Psychosocial and cognitive aspects. In S. Feinstein et al. (Eds.), *Adolescent psychiatry: Developmental and clinical studies* (Vol. 9). Chicago: University of Chicago Press.

Pfeffer, C. (1981). The family system of suicidal children. *American Journal of Psychotherapy, 35,* 330-341.

Pokorny, A. D. (1975). Self-destruction and the automobile. In A. Roberts (Ed.), *Self-destructive behavior.* Springfield, IL: Charles C Thomas.

Preventing teenage suicide: Everyone can help. (1983, June 2). *Christian Science Monitor,* p. B-1.

Ray, L., & Johnson, N. (1983). Adolescent suicide. *The Personnel and Guidance Journal, 162*, 131-135.

Roberts, A. R. (1975). *Self-destructive behavior.* Springfield, IL: Charles C Thomas.

Robin, A. L., & Foster, S. L. (1984). Problem-solving communication training: A behavioral family systems approach to parent-adolescent conflict. In P. Karoly & J. Steffen (Eds.), *Adolescent behavior disorders: Foundations and contemporary concerns.* Lexington, MA: Lexington Books.

Rosenblatt, J. (1981). Youth suicide. *Editorial Research Reports, 1*, 431-438.

Rosenkrantz, A. L. (1978). A note on adolescent suicide: Incidence, dynamics, and some suggestions for treatment. *Adolescence, 13*, 209-213.

Rosenthal, M. J. (1981). Sexual differences in the suicidal behavior of young people. In S. Feinstein et al (Eds.), *Adolescent psychiatry: Developmental and clinical studies* (Vol. 9). Chicago: University of Chicago Press.

Ross, C. (1980). Mobilizing schools for suicide prevention. *Suicide and Life Threatening Behavior, 10*, 239-243.

Sanborn, D. E., Sanborn, C., & Cimbolic, P. (1973). Two years of suicide: A study of adolescent suicide in New Hampshire. *Child Psychiatry and Human Development, 3*, 234-242.

Sartore, R. L. (1976). Students and suicide: An interpersonal tragedy. *Theory into Practice, 15*, 337-339.

Shaffer, D., & Fisher, P. (1981). The epidemiology of suicide in young children and adolescents. *Journal of the American Academy of Child Psychiatry, 20*, 545-565.

Smith, D. (1976). Adolescent suicide: A problem for teachers? *Phi Delta Kappa, 57*, 539-542.

Smith, E. J. (1981). Adolescent suicide: A growing problem for the school and family. *Urban Education, 16*, 279-296.

Swenson, B., & Rabin, P. (1981). Teenage suicide attempts and parental divorce. *New England Journal of Medicine, 304*, 1048.

Tabachnick, N. (1981). The interlocking psychologies of suicide and adolescence. In S. Feinstein et al. (Eds.), *Adolescent psychiatry: Developmental and clinical studiese* (Vol. 9). Chicago: University of Chicago Press.

Tishler, C. L. (1982). Parental negative self and adolescent suicide attempts. *Journal of the American Academy of Child Psychiatry, 21*, 404.

Tishler, C. L., & Jacobs, L. A. (1983). Making life meaningful for youth: Preventing suicide. In L. Arnold (Ed.), *Preventing adolescent alienation.* Lexington, MA: D. C. Heath.

Tishler, C. L., & McKenry, P. C. (1982). Parental negative self and adolescent suicide attempts. *Journal of the American Academy of Child Psychiatry, 21*, 404-408.

Tishler, C. L., & McKenry, P. C. (1983). Intrapsychic symptom dimensions of adolescent suicide attempters. *Journal of Family Practice, 16*, 731-734.

Toolan, J. M. (1975). Suicide in children and adolescents. *American Journal of Psychotherapy, 29*, 339-344.

Topol, P., & Reznikoff, M. (1982). Perceived peer and family relationships, hopelessness and locus of control as factors in adolescent suicide attempts. *Suicide & Life Threatening Behavior, 12*, 141-150.

Uber, S. R. (1983). Perceived family system of the adolescent suicide attempter. *Dissertation Abstracts International, 43*(Sec. B), 2362-2363.

U. S. Congress, Senate, Committee on Judiciary, Subcommittee on Juvenile Justice. (1984a, October). *Hearings on teenage suicide* (Testimony by A. L. Berman on behalf of the American Psychological Association).

U. S. Congress, Senate, Committee on Judiciary, Subcommittee on Juvenile Justice. (1984b, October). *Hearings on teenage suicide* (Testimony by M. Herbert on Teenage Suicide in a Public School System).

U. S. vital statistics, 1974 & 1975, Volume II—Mortality. (1978). Washington, DC: National Center for Health Statistics.

Walch, S. M. (1977). Adolescent attempted suicide: Analysis of the differences in male and female suicidal behavior. *Dissertation Abstracts International, 38*(Sec. B), 2892-2893.

Wattenberg, E. (1986). The fate of baby boomers and their children. *Social Work, 58,* 20-28.

Wenz, F. (1979). Self-injury behavior, economic status and the family anomic syndrome among adolescents. *Adolescence, 14,* 387-398.

Wodarski, J. S. (1982). Single parents and children: A review for social workers. *Family Therapy, 9,* 311-320.

Wodarski, J. S. (1987). A social learning theory approach to teaching adolescents about drinking and driving: A multiple variable follow-up evaluation. *Journal of Behavior Therapy and Experimental Psychiatry, 18,* 51-60.

Wodarski, J. S., & Hedrick, M. (1987). Violent children: A practice paradigm. *Social Work in Education, 10,* 28-42.

World health statistics annual 1972: Vital statistics and causes of death (Vol. 1). (1975). Geneva: World Health Organization.

Chapter 7

VIOLENT CHILDREN: A PRACTICE PARADIGM

By John S. Wodarski and Mitzi Hedrick

FOR THE PAST several decades, the number of youths involved in violent crimes has increased. Additionally, the number of youths involved in violent crimes at an earlier age is increasing. In 1978, for example, the *Uniform Crime Reports* indicated that nearly two million youths under age 18 were charged with an offense. Of these, 58,593 were serious offenses such as murder or non-negligent manslaughter, forcible rape, robbery, and aggravated assault. More than 700,000 of the charged youths were under age 15 and 79,007 were 10 years old or under (U. S. Department of Justice, 1979, p. 193).

Between 1969 and 1978 arrests of males under age 18 increased by 10.1 percent for most types of offenses. In general, the rate of violent crime rose by 40.6 percent. In 1974, 1,683,000 youths under age 18 were arrested for violent crimes, compared with 2,279,000 in 1978. Although the proportion of youths in U. S. society varies over the years, delinquency rates for youths remain high (Baker & Rubel, 1980; Blyth, Thiel, Bush, & Simmons, 1978; Rubel, 1978).

In 1983, almost 1,000 juveniles were arrested for murder, almost 3,000 for rape, and more than 19,000 for aggravated assault. These arrest statistics underestimate the number of offenses committed. Research also demonstrates that among the small group of juvenile offenders that commit these crimes, a substantial proportion continue to commit crimes as adults (Hamparian, Davis, Jacobson, & McGraw, 1985).

In an attempt to combat the problem, researchers have explored every theoretical focus, from social to neurological, related to antisocial

135

behavior of youths. Because a large number of background factors, such as unemployment, peer association, stress, low socioeconomic status, marital problems, physical problems, and type of neighborhood, is posited to contribute to the problem, researchers often feel that in focusing on a single aspect of the problem, validity, accuracy, and real-life applicability are lost (Feldman, Caplinger, & Wodarski, 1983; Gibbons, 1986).

Providing services to potentially violent children has been a major focus of social work practice. Various theories, such as psychoanalytic and behavioral, have attempted to explain violent behavior. Additionally, a variety of treatment modalities, such as intensive individual, group, residential treatment and family therapy, has been proposed to address the problem (Curry, 1985). Recent research indicates that violent children are one of the most troublesome groups in terms of service provision (Kazdin, 1985, 1987). The problems of violent children are not resolved by current interventions and are costly interventions in terms of length of incarceration and service expenditures. Moreover, if not helped, this group of relatively few chronic offenders are responsible for a disproportionate number of crimes.

The concept of violent behavior is vague. In this chapter, the authors focus on those acts that are of greatest concern to social workers: violent behavior that involves the intent to do physical harm to other individuals — specifically rape, murder and physical assault.

AGE OF ONSET AND FREQUENCY OF VIOLENT BEHAVIOR

Data indicate that the earlier the age of an adolescent's first arrest, the greater the probability of future violence. For example, one study found that when the first arrest age was between ages 8 and 10 years, the mean number of violent offenses for an individual was .25. Likewise, the incidences for ages 11 to 13 was .24; for ages 14 to 16, .22; for ages 17 to 19, .11; for ages 20 to 22, .04; and for ages 23 to 25, .03. Furthermore, 20 percent of those classified as recidivists by age 18 were involved in violent crime as adults (Guttridge, Mednick, & Van Dusen, 1983).

Violent offenders tend to commit more crimes than do other offenders. Moreover, as an adolescent commits more offenses, it becomes more likely that the offenses will be violent. Of the men charged with 18 or more offenses, about 10 percent have committed at least one violent act (Guttridge et al., 1983). Furthermore, while all other index offense types (such as robbery) either decrease or are unaffected by age, violence shows an increase with age. Wolfgang, Figlio and Sellin (1972) showed an increase of 21 percent in violent crimes committed from ages 10 and under to age 17.

There is evidence of the development of a criminal career over time, which can lead to the commission of a violent crime. Thus, there is a substantial link between juvenile crime and adult crime. Data suggest that the violent offender is a chronic adult criminal or recidivist who began committing crimes at an early age, possibly as early as age eight, who engages in a high number of crimes, and who commits a wide variety of crimes. A small proportion of violent chronic offenders accounts for a large proportion of all arrests (Farrington & Tarling, 1985).

CRITICAL VARIABLES IN THE DEVELOPMENT OF VIOLENT BEHAVIOR

Child Management

The most significant variable in the development of violent behavior appears to be lack of appropriate parenting. For example, parental laxness (lack of monitoring or discipline) is significantly correlated with delinquency (Wilson, 1980). Families classified as lax were likely to have a delinquency rate more than seven times that of the families classified as strict. Likewise, Patterson and Stouthamer-Loeber (1984) found significant correlations between the measures of parent monitoring and discipline and a variety of delinquent behaviors. Loeber (1982) posited that chronically violent youth are found in homes where parental management skills are disrupted chronically or where the children are overmonitored or not monitored sufficiently. Parental aggression, lack of supervision, conflict, and lack of maternal affection all contribute to criminal behavior, according to a study by McCord (1979). Furthermore, the study suggested that these variables contributed more to the criminal behavior of adults than did aggressive behavior exhibited as youths.

Additional data indicate that violent children usually come from violent families. The theory is that violent children observe parents resolve conflict by violent means and learn to solve their own conflicts in this way. Violence is thus modeled as a problem-solving strategy. Violent children also have a history of non-compliant behavior—that is, they do not respond to reasonable requests by parents. Such coercive behaviors subsequently are reinforced, and the children learn coercive means of solving problems (Kazdin, 1985). When children start school, coercive behaviors accelerate toward parents and, at school, toward prosocial peers and adults.

Cognitive, Social and Academic Skills: Contributing Factors

Because of their coercive behaviors, violent children do not learn empathic behaviors nor adequate cognitive strategies for dealing with anger. Likewise, they do not learn to handle stress in a prosocial manner. Thus, violent children are not prepared adequately to deal with stress once they leave protected homes.

Dishion, Loeber, Stouthamer-Loeber, and Patterson (1984) found that academic skills deficits in the areas of verbal intelligence, reading achievement, homework completion, and mother's rating of school competence correlated most significantly with violence in adolescents. Rejection by adults and prosocial peers at school has been related significantly to violent behavior (Kaplan & Robbins, 1983). Patterson (1982) postulated that the lack of social or academic skills increases the child's chance of failure in school and with peers and family and thus exacerbates the child's alienation from prosocial relationships.

In addition, there is positive association between dropping out of high school and later criminality (Thornberry, Moore, & Christenson, 1985). Family rejection furthers the adoption of deviant responses and is associated positively with long-term criminality (Patterson & Dishion, 1985).

Self-Esteem and Peer Relations

The literature indicates that violent individuals have poor self-concepts and difficulty integrating with prosocial peer groups. Difficulties at school and rejection and abuse by parents tend to reduce self-esteem among these youth. In addition, violent individuals usually are physically unattractive, which contributes to poor self-esteem and rejection by peers (Agnew, 1984; Hanson, Henggeler, Haefele, & Rodick, 1984).

Violent individuals usually are not in the mainstream of prosocial peer culture. They do not form attachments to prosocial institutions of society and, instead, are part of a small group of peers who reinforce each other for violent behaviors. In the view of Hirschi's control theory (1969), youth who lack adequate attachments to school and parents are "free" to engage in delinquent behavior. Delinquent peers have been found to support participation in delinquent acts through positive reinforcement (Patterson & Dishion, 1985).

Findings in one study showed that parent reports of strong participation in a delinquent peer group most consistently predicted serious and repeated arrests among adolescent males (Hanson et al., 1984). Indeed, association with delinquent peers was found to be most prevalent among those youths officially classified as delinquents by law enforcement agencies (Grove & Crutchfield, 1982). Analyses strongly suggest that membership in a delinquent peer group is a strong predictor of subsequent increases in violent behavior (Elliott, Ageton, & Canter, 1979; Patterson & Dishion, 1985).

Alcohol seems to be a critical influence later in the process of the development of violent behavior. Violent adolescents cannot process cognitively, nor can they manage stress. Alcohol reduces inhibitions and facilitates aggressive responses (Collins, 1981). An available weapon also increases the potential for violent behavior; usually, if a weapon is available, violent children eventually will use the weapon to reduce stress or to resolve conflict. Violent children therefore are at great risk in communities where weapons are readily available (Wolfgang & Weiner, 1982).

Developmental Process

Home Environment. Evidence has shown that children who engage in antisocial behavior can be grouped as "stealers" and "aggressors." Which type of antisocial behavior a child engages in is determined in large part by the type of parental supervision exercised (Hewitt & Jenkins, 1946; Loeber & Schmaling, 1985; Patterson, 1982). Stealers come from homes with insufficient monitoring and discipline, whereas aggressors come from homes in which parenting is characterized by more aversive interaction. The child's age also determines the type of antisocial activity in which the child engages. A younger child who hits playmates over the head with a toy may later fistfight and, having gained entry into a gang, may be introduced to stealing. The authors posit that these behaviors fall on a continuum, which if left unattended will increase in frequency, range of contexts in which the behavior is exhibited, variety, and severity.

Childhood Crime. Robins and Ratcliff (1979) found that early aggression, theft and lying are associated with later delinquency. For example, 39 percent of the children who had been involved in three or more types of antisocial behavior became delinquent, compared to only 6 percent of the children with a single type of antisocial behavior. Shapland (1978) measured 48 types of behavior and their frequency in a self-reported delinquency study of adolescents aged 11 to 14. Petty offenses were committed at all ages; however, the more serious acts were committed at later ages. The number of the types of crimes committed increased with age, and the boys who committed the largest number of offenses also committed a more varied range of offenses.

The type of violent behavior that a child displays is a product of the parental management techniques exercised or not exercised, the age of the child, and the child's involvement in antisocial behaviors. The higher the rate at which the child participates in antisocial behaviors, the greater the child's potential for entrance into a career of violence. Thus, there is evidence to support a quantitative development of violent behavior. Certain researchers present data suggesting that potentially violent youths are overtly antisocial at preschool age (Loeber & Schmaling, 1985).

Transition to Adult Crime. Data suggest that exhibition of antisocial and delinquent behavior is a sound basis for predicting future problems. In a study of violent criminals in London, McClintock (as cited by Hood & Sparks, 1970) found that violent recidivists had previous convictions for non-violent crimes. Violent offenders, more than other offenders, tend to commit more crimes, and those who commit many offenses are more likely to be violent (Guttridge et al., 1983). Furthermore, there may be a tendency for these offenders to commit more serious crimes as they get older (Farrington & Tarling, 1985).

Moreover, the data indicate that juvenile delinquent activities often are followed by adult crime. Farrington (1983) shows a close relationship between juvenile and adult convictions. In addition, more chronic offenders as a group committed the greatest proportion of crimes, and those chronic offenders were identified as the youths first convicted at the earliest ages.

PROFILE OF VIOLENT YOUTHS

Having established a category of children who appear to be most at risk for entrance into an environment conducive to committing a violent act, the next logical step is to attempt to identify the children in that category most likely to actually commit violent acts.

In a study by Loeber and Schmaling (1985) that compared fighters, stealers and versatile youths (children who fight **and** steal), the versatile youths scored the highest, meaning they committed the greatest variety of crimes, in almost all delinquent acts. Furthermore, the versatile youths had a higher rate of association with delinquent peer groups, had a more negative outlook on life, and were more hyperactive and disobedient. The versatile youths came from homes with the poorest parental management techniques and were the most disturbed on measures of family processes, specifically lack of monitoring; inconsistent rule application; poor supervision, reasoning, and communication; and rejection by the mother.

Patterson (1982) found that similarities and differences between fighters and stealers include non-compliance, arrested socialization (maximizes immediate gains at someone else's expense, lack of impulse control); reduced responsiveness to social stimuli (unresponsive to ordinary social reinforcers and to threats and scolding, attentional deficits); and skills deficits (academic achievement, work, peer relations).

Violent youths typically have low IQs and assaultive tendencies, such as instigating fights and defying authority, and exhibit cruelty and malicious mischief. They are depressed and frustrated, feel inadequate, lack internal inhibitions, and expect immediate gratification. Violent youths more often come from low-income neighborhoods, witness violent acts, and are subjected to parental abuse (although not necessarily physical abuse) (Brown, 1975). Rejection and aggressive behavior are modeled in the home, which most likely is headed by a single parent (Lefkowitz, Eron, Walder, & Huesmann, 1977).

Model of Prevention

Treatment

The authors believe that early identification and intervention based on empirical knowledge with youths exhibiting high rates of antisocial behavior would be most instrumental in preventing delinquency.

Parents must be taught adequate parenting skills, with emphasis on communication. This approach should alleviate the deleterious circumstances that affect potentially violent children. These children can be identified by an inflated rate of antisocial behavior or through contact with the law. Children must be taught life skills in the following areas: cognitive anger control, problem solving, peer enhancement, and substance abuse education (Feindler & Ecton, 1986; Kaplan, Konecni, & Novaco, 1984; Spence & Marzillier, 1981). By introducing interventions at both home and school, it can be determined which is most effective, either singularly or in combination, in helping aggressive youngsters overcome their antisocial tendencies.

Preventive Paradigm Components

Treatment is proposed for antisocial children characterized by their rates of preschool and early elementary school non-compliant activity; restlessness; impulsivity; coercive exchanges with parents, siblings and peers; and aggression. Data indicate that if intervention does not occur during this period, the probability is increased that the behaviors will be chronic (Wolf, Braukmann, & Ramp, 1987). Groups are used as the focus of service delivery.

Behavioral Group Work Approach. Despite the growing emphasis on group work intervention recently, relatively few clients are treated in this manner as compared with those treated individually. Services provided to children in groups offer several positive aspects:

(1) The group interaction typifies many kinds of daily interactions. Services that facilitate behaviors that enable people to interact in groups are likely to better prepare them for participation in larger society; that is, the interaction will help them learn social skills necessary to secure reinforcement (Feldman & Wodarski, 1975).

(2) If a behavior is learned in a group context, it is likely to come under the control of a greater number of discriminative stimuli; therefore, greater generalization of the behavior can occur for a broader variety of interactional contexts.

(3) Groups provide a context in which behaviors can be tested in a realistic atmosphere; that is, clients can get immediate peer feedback on their problem-solving behaviors. Likewise, they are provided with role models to facilitate acquisition of requisite social behavior.

(4) Groups provide a more valid locus for accurate diagnosis and a more potent means for changing client behavior (Meyer & Smith, 1977; Rose, 1977).

(5) The provision of services through groups greatly increases the number of clients who can be served.

(6) Groups provide peer support for altered prosocial behavior; children can practice and receive reinforcement for new social skills, which facilitates their acquisition. These skills in turn enhance peer relationships and increase clients' satisfaction with life.

Social workers should be trained to incorporate basic social learning principles that can be used in working with adolescents in groups (Feldman & Wodarski, 1975; Wodarski, Feldman, & Flax, 1972). Treatment objectives can be achieved through contingency contracts, positive reinforcement (to encourage preadolescents to change their behaviors); modeling relevant requisite behaviors; and structuring reinforcements (such as approval) that the group members can provide themselves. The comprehensive program consists of a family and school intervention in the fourth, fifth, and sixth grades. The school intervention consists of four major components: (1) cognitive anger control, (2) problem solving, (3) peer skills development, and (4) substance abuse education.

Cognitive Anger Control. Violent individuals lack the means to control anger (LeCroy, 1983). Professionals must be prepared to help preadolescents develop the following skills:

(1) Identify stresses that can provoke anger and subsequent violent behavior.

(2) Develop cognitive relaxation skills to reduce the effects of stresses.

(3) Learn how to receive assertive statements and deal with the anger of others.

(4) Develop appropriate communication and assertion skills.

(5) Practice alternate behavior, such as stimulus removal, in anger-provoking situations.

Problem Solving. Preadolescents who have difficulty coping with the daily problems of living should be taught a problem-solving approach based on the work of D'Zurilla and Goldfried (1971), Goldfried and Goldfried (1975), Schinke and Gilchrist (1984) and Spivack and Shure (1974). The skills emphasized are how to generate information, how to generate possible solutions, how to evaluate possible courses of action, and how to choose and implement strategies by understanding how certain consequences and stimuli can control problem-solving behavior, isolating and defining a behavior to be changed, using stimulus control techniques to influence rates of problem-solving behavior, and using appropriate consequences to increase or decrease a behavior.

Peer Enhancement. Altering dissatisfaction about interpersonal relationships and the youths' perception of themselves as lacking in social skills is important in preventing violence. Thus, potentially violent children must learn how to interact with others in meaningful and satisfying ways. Facets of the program developed by Lange and Jakubowski (1976) are proposed, involving conversational skills training, use of appropriate non-verbal communication, and development of assertive behavior to decrease stress produced by inadequately met social needs.

Specific skills taught include how to introduce one's self, how to initiate and continue conversations, how to give and receive compliments, how to enhance appearance, how to make and refuse requests, how to express feelings spontaneously, and how to use appropriate non-verbal behavior to enhance sociability.

Substance Abuse. Substance abuse is the last link in establishing a violent career and is a major factor in maintaining it (Collins, 1981). Thus, children should participate in a program designed to educate them about drugs and how substance abuse issues apply to their own lives. The program should emphasize acquisition of self-management skills.

Basic Knowledge About Drug Consumption and Usage. Children must learn about drug use, including what dosage of drugs a body can absorb in a given period, and when an intoxicated person is in an emergency situation. They should also learn how to deal with such an occurrence, the physiological affects of drugs, the amount of alcohol in alcoholic beverages, and how to assess a drug problem.

Self-Management and Maintenance. Children should be taught basic principles of social learning theory to enable them to manage situations involving drugs. Social learning theorists emphasize that drug abuse is learned from the consequences of drug use. These consequences most often include stress reduction (lessened inhibition in sociability around peers); removal from an unpleasant situation (because adolescents tend to consume more drugs at one sitting than adults, this behavior more often results in their passing out); and an excuse for otherwise unacceptable behavior (for example, aggressive or flirtatious behavior might be excused) (Wodarski, 1987).

Role-Play Simulation Exercises. Role-play simulation exercises can be used to help children practice refusing drugs in a socially acceptable manner within normal peer contexts (Foy et al., 1976). Children can develop more effective ways of dealing with social pressures to consume drugs. Specific situations can be practiced in which individuals apply pressure to others to consume excessive amounts of drugs. Children practice reactions to statements like: "One drink won't hurt you"; "What kind of friend are you"; or "Just have a little one, I'll make sure you won't have any more."

Family Prevention Strategy

Parents likewise must be educated about the dynamics of violent behavior. Parents must be taught problem-solving and communication skills for conflict resolution (Robin & Foster, 1984). The five steps involved in problem-solving should be delineated: (1) problem definition, (2) generation of alternate solutions, (3) decision making, (4) planning solution implementation, and (5) renegotiation. Parents then discuss these steps in the group and role play how to use the procedures. During the role play, group members attempt to solve problems of adolescents of other group members.

Information on use of positive and negative control with adolescents should be included. The focus within this material is on increasing use of positive reinforcement for appropriate behavior rather than the often used coercive processes such as negative reinforcement and punishment (Forehand & McMahon, 1981; Patterson, 1981).

Parents should understand that better communication skills, problem-solving skills, and positive reinforcement will result in a better parent-child relationship and will reduce the probability of violent behavior. Additional sessions should be scheduled to support the use of these practices and to refine their implementation.

SUMMARY

The effectiveness of an interdisciplinary approach to the identification and prediction of, and intervention with, antisocial, delinquent, and potentially violent youth cannot be measured easily. Given the proven ineffectiveness of previous treatments, however, this approach should be attempted.

With increased awareness of the warning signs of violent behavior, intervention in the home on a more personal, day-to-day basis might take place. Education about how to identify the warning signals and how to teach parenting skills is also necessary. Because parents and peers are primary influences on violent behavior, prevention efforts should be directed toward these two groups. Models for such programs are available. This intervention is ambitious, yet it has the potential to produce significant steps toward alleviating the problem of antisocial youths.

The authors have reviewed theoretical knowledge and research about violent children. Factors that affect the development of violent behavior in children were elaborated. A prevention paradigm that uses a family-school intervention in the late elementary school years was proposed as the treatment of choice.

REFERENCES

Agnew, R. (1984). Appearance and delinquency. *Criminology, 22*(3), 421-440.

Baker, K., & Rubel, R. (Eds.). (1980). *Violence and crimes in the schools.* Lexington, MA: D. C. Heath & Co.

Blyth, D. A., Thiel, K. S., Bush, D., & Simmons, R. G. (1978). *Another look at school crime: Student as victim.* Boys Town, NE: Center for the Study of Youth Development. (mimeograph)

Brown, S. (1975). Social class, child maltreatment, and delinquent behavior. *Criminology, 22*(2), 259-278.

Collins, J. J. (1981). *Alcohol use and criminal behavior: An executive summary.* Washington, DC: U. S. Department of Justice, National Institute of Justice.

Curry, J. F. (1985). Aggressive or delinquent adolescents: Family therapy interventions. *Practice Applications, 3*(1).

Dishion, T. J., Loeber, R., Stouthamer-Loeber, M., & Patterson, G. R. (1984). Skills deficits and male adolescent delinquency. *Journal of Abnormal Child Psychology, 12*, 37-54.

D'Zurilla, T. J., & Goldfried, M. R. (1971). Problem-solving and behavior modification. *Journal of Abnormal Psychology, 78*, 107-126.

Elliott, D. S., Ageton, S. S., & Canter, R. J. (1979). An integrated theoretical perspective on delinquent behavior. *Journal of Research in Crime and Delinquency, 16*, 3-27.

Farrington, D. P. (1983). Offending from 10 to 25 years of age. In K. Van Dusen & S. Mednick (Eds.), *Prospective studies of crime and delinquency.* Boston: Kluwer-Nijhoff.

Farrington, D. P., & Tarling, R. (Eds.). (1985). *Prediction in criminology.* Albany: State University of New York Press.

Feindler, E. L., & Ecton, R. B. (1986). *Adolescent anger control: Cognitive-behavioral techniques.* New York: Pergamon Press.

Feldman, R. A., Caplinger, T. E., & Wodarski, J. S. (1983). *The St. Louis conundrum: The effective treatment of antisocial youths.* Englewood Cliffs, NJ: Prentice-Hall.

Feldman, R. A., & Wodarski, J. S. (1975). *Contemporary approaches to group treatment.* San Francisco: Jossey-Bass.

Forehand, R., & McMahon, R. J. (1981). *Helping the noncompliant child: A clinician's guide to parent training.* New York: Guilford.

Foy, C. W., Miller, P. M., Eisler, R. M., & O'Toole, O. H. (1976). Social skills training to teach alcoholics to refuse drinks effectively. *Journal of Studies on Alcohol, 37*(9), 1340-1345.

Gibbons, D. C. (1986). Juvenile delinquency: Can social science find a cure? *Crime & Delinquency, 32*(2), 186-204.

Goldfried, M., & Goldfried, A. (1975). Cognitive change methods. In F. Kanfer & A. Goldstein (Eds.), *Helping people change.* New York: Pergamon Press.

Grove, W. R., & Crutchfield, R. D. (1982). The family and juvenile delinquency. *The Sociological Quarterly, 23,* 301-319.

Guttridge, P., Mednick, S. A., & Van Dusen, K. (1983). Criminal violence in a birth cohort. In K. Van Dusen & S. Mednick (Eds.), *Prospective studies of crime and delinquency.* Boston: Kluwer-Nijhoff.

Hamparian, D. M., Davis, J. M., Jacobson, J. M., & McGraw, R. E. (1985). *The young criminal years of the violent few.* Washington, DC: U. S. Department of Justice, Office of Juvenile Justice and Delinquency Prevention.

Hanson, C. L., Henggeler, S. W., Haefele, W. F., & Rodick, J. D. (1984). Demographic, individual, family relationship correlates of serious and repeated crime among adolescents and their siblings. *Journal of Consulting and Clinical Psychology, 52*(4), 528-538.

Hewitt, L. E., & Jenkins, R. L. (1946). *Fundamental patterns of maladjustment: The dynamics of their origin.* Michigan Child Guidance Institute.

Hirschi, T. (1969). *Causes of delinquency.* Berkeley: University of California Press.

Hood, R., & Sparks, R. (1970). *Key issues in criminology.* London: Weindelfeld & Nicholson.

Kaplan, H. B., & Robbins, C. (1983). Testing a general theory of deviant behavior in longitudinal perspective. In K. Van Dusen & S. Mednick (Eds.), *Prospective studies of crime and delinquency.* Boston, MA: Kluwer-Nijhoff.

Kaplan, R. M., Konecni, V. J., & Novaco, R. W. (Eds.), (1984). *Aggression in children and youth* (NATO Advanced Science Institute Series, Behavioural and Social Sciences, No. 17). The Hague, The Netherlands: Martinus Nijhoff.

Kazdin, A. E. (1985). *Treatment of antisocial behavior in children and adolescents: Alternative interventions and their effectiveness.* Homewood, IL: Dorsey Press.

Kazdin, A. E. (1987). Treatment of antisocial behavior in children: Current status and future directions. *Psychological Bulletin, 102*(2), 187-203.

Lange, A. J., & Jakubowski, P. (1976). *Responsible assertive behavior.* Champaign, IL: Research Press.

LeCroy, C. W. (1983). Social-cognitive group work with children. *Behavior Group Therapy, 5*(1), 91-116.

Lefkowitz, M., Eron, L., Walder, L., & Huesmann, L. R. (1977). *Growing up to be violent: A longitudinal study of the development of aggression.* New York: Pergamon.

Loeber, R. (1982). The stability of antisocial and delinquent child behavior: A review. *Child Development, 53,* 1431-1446.

Loeber, R., & Schmaling, K. B. (1985). The utility of differentiating between mixed and pure forms of antisocial child behavior. *Journal of Abnormal Child Psychology, 13*(2), 315-336.

McCord, J. (1979). Some child-rearing antecedents of criminal behavior in adult men. *Journal of Personality and Social Psychology, 37*(9), 1477-1486.

Meyer, R. G., & Smith, S. S. (1977). A crisis in group therapy. *American Psychologist, 32,* 638-643.

Patterson, G. R. (1981). *Coercive family process.* Eugene, OR: Castalia.

Patterson, G. R. (1982). *Coercive family process* (Vol. 3). Eugene, OR: Castalia.

Patterson, G. R., & Dishion, T. J. (1985). Contributions of families and peers to delinquency. *Criminology, 23*(1), 63-79.

Patterson, G. R., & Stouthamer-Loeber, M. (1984). The correlation of family management practices and delinquency. *Child Development, 55,* 1299-1307.

Robin, A. L., & Foster, S. L. (1984). Problem-solving communication training: A behavioral family systems approach to parent-adolescent conflict. In P. Karoly & J. Steffen (Eds.), *Adolescent behavior disorders: Foundations and contemporary concerns* (pp. 195-240). Lexington, MA: D. C. Heath.

Robins, L. N., & Ratcliff, K. S. (1979). Risk factors in the continuation of childhood antisocial behavior into adulthood. *International Journal of Mental Health, 7,* 96-116.

Rose, S. D. (1977). *Group therapy: A behavioral approach.* Englewood Cliffs, NJ: Prentice-Hall.

Rubel, R. J. (1978). Analysis and critique of HEW's *Safe school study report to Congress. Crime and Delinquency, 24,* 257-265.

Schinke, S. P., & Gilchrist, L. D. (1984). *Life skills counseling with adolescents.* Baltimore: University Park Press.

Shapland, J. M. (1978). Self-reported delinquency in boys age 11 to 14. *British Journal of Criminology, 18*(3), 255-266.

Spence, S. H., & Marzillier, J. S. (1981). Social skills training with adolescent male offenders: II. Short term, long-term and generalized effects. *Behaviour Research and Therapy, 19*(4), 349-368.

Spivack, G., & Shure, M. B. (1974). *Social adjustment of young children.* San Francisco: Jossey-Bass.

Thornberry, T. P., Moore, M., & Christenson, R. L. (1985). The effect of dropping out of high school on subsequent criminal behavior. *Criminology, 23*(1), 3-18.

U. S. Department of Justice. (1979). *Uniform crime reports, 1979.* Washington, DC: U. S. Government Printing Office.

Wilson, H. (1980). Parental supervision: A neglected aspect of delinquency. *The British Journal of Criminology, 20*(3), 203-235.

Wodarski, J. S. (1987). Evaluating a social learning approach to teaching adolescents about alcohol and driving: A multiple variable evaluation. *Journal of Social Service Research, 10*(2/3/4), 121-144.

Wodarski, J. S., Feldman, R. A., & Flax, N. (1972). Social learning theory in group work practice with antisocial children. *Clinical Social Work Journal, 1*(2), 78-93.

Wolf, M. M., Braukmann, C. J., & Ramp, K. A. (1987). Serious delinquent behavior as a part of a significantly handicapping condition: Cures and supporting environments. *Journal of Applied Behavior Analysis, 20,* 347-359.

Wolfgang, M. E., Figlio, R. M., & Sellin, T. (1972). *Delinquency in a birth cohort.* Chicago, IL: University of Chicago Press.

Wolfgang, M. E., & Weiner, N. A. (Eds.). (1982). *Criminal violence.* Beverly Hills: Sage Publications.

Chapter 8

COMPREHENSIVE EMPLOYMENT PREPARATION FOR ADOLESCENTS WITH DEVELOPMENTAL DISABILITIES: AN EMPIRICAL PARADIGM

The passage of a young person from adolescence to adulthood is marked by a number of events. Of these, none is more important than the young person's finding work and becoming economically independent. Today in the United States, this transition is often painful and frustrating, and large numbers of youth are failing to achieve it. (Dayton, 1981, p. 321).

IT IS CRITICAL to note the importance Americans place on employment and financial security. The Gallup organization (1980) conducted a study of adults in 1977 and another in 1980 and reported that the two most important problems facing their families at that time were economic and financial security employment. There is substantial research, for example, that indicates that for the majority of individuals, work is the single most defining aspect of living in American society. Coles (1976) discovered that work was the most significant measure of "grown-up" status among working-class people.

Work has special meaning to the psychosocial development of young people with developmental disabilities (Canonico & Lombardi, 1984; Ferguson & Ferguson, 1986). It is an opportunity to establish one's own identity, to gain independence, to contribute to family finances, to acquire prestige, and to try out adult roles. Conversely, unemployment at this age lowers feelings of self-esteem, and long spells of joblessness may precipitate catastrophic psychological problems and dependency. In Briar's study (1976) of youths, the impact of unemployment made them feel like they were "going crazy" and "suffocating." Some felt "mad at the whole world," "useless," "fed up," "stranded," and "incompetent and a failure." In addition to being bored, frightened, insecure, depressed and confused, some of them claimed their joblessness caused them to have problems with alcohol, eating and sleeping. Increases in family conflicts also were reported. There are also indications that drug addiction, teenage pregnancy and family violence are related to youth joblessness (Dayton, 1978; Greenberger & Steinberg, 1986).

Although the literature indicates that work does enhance one's mental health, it also points out that many youths, particularly those with developmental disabilities, are motivated to work but lack "know-how" about how to accurately assess their own interests and abilities, plan for employment, and find and hold jobs. Many youth, especially those with negative school experiences, may suffer from alienation from society and a lack of self-esteem. For youth who are developmentally disabled to be successfully employed, data suggest that it is necessary to take a holistic approach but also preparing the youth both psychologically and socially for the job market.

This chapter elucidates strategies for facilitating the preparation of high-risk developmentally disabled youth populations for work. Community-based strategies include vocational enrichment programs; pursuing, securing and maintaining employment; social skills; cognitive anger control; problem-solving; and interpersonal skills.

Historical Review

For over 60 years, conventional rehabilitation programs have focused on helping people with disabilities who had potential vocational prospects. Traditionally, to be eligible for services, a client must be considered to have a reasonable expectation in terms of employability. In the 1970s, however, new laws (P.L. 94-482, 93-112, and 95-602) made provisions and arrangements for increasing rehabilitation services to a wider range of handicapped individuals. Under new laws, most of the provisions and arrangements are simply an extension or amplification of existing rehabilitation practices. All categories of mental retardation and other developmental disabilities, such as cerebral palsy, epilepsy, autism, and other conditions closely related to mental retardation, are eligible for appropriate services, whether or not a potential vocational goal is possible (Riggar, 1979).

Vocational education is usually delivered by colleges, technical institutes, and community rehabilitation facilities. Data indicate most workers are placed in janitorial and kitchen jobs. These positions, characterized by easy acquisition and high turnover, are the most available and the least difficult to develop. Other employment possibilities that are usually considered in vocational education include: computer operator, health aide, housekeeper, office worker, auto mechanic, switchboard operator, order processing clerk, laundry operator, drill operator, printed-circuit assembler, packager, machinery and mechanical operations worker.

In spite of new legislation and emphasis on employment among the private sector and the government, a very small fraction of the severely and profoundly disabled people are employed in the nation's labor force. The United States Commission on Civil Rights in 1983 reported that between 50 percent and 80 percent of all persons with disabilities are unemployed. For example, less than 12 percent of all *severely* disabled individuals were employed in Virginia and all of them were underemployed (Wehman, Kregel, & Zoller, 1984).

Data indicate that 75 percent of physically disabled and 90 percent of mentally disabled youth could work competitively or in sheltered employment. However, lack of social preparation for employment is cited frequently as the cause for unemployment (Coughran & Daniels, 1983). Too frequently, disabled youth who have reached employable age (16 or above) are referred to state rehabilitation agencies and are then determined to be ineligible for service because of lack of previous social preparation (Goldberg, 1981). If disabled youths are placed, data suggest that a majority are terminated within six months in their jobs due to inappropriate social behavior. Frequently listed are maladaptive behaviors, including non-compliance, off-task, bizarre, aggressive, stereotyped, self-destructive, etc.; extreme dependence on direct supervision; inappropriate interaction with supervisor and co-workers; excessive tardiness; inadequate attendance; insufficient speed and accuracy; failure to notify employer when unable to report to work; unacceptable personal appearance; transportation difficulties; and so forth (Karan & Knight, 1983; Shafer, 1987).

Most state rehabilitation agencies have focused on vocational aspects such as specific work skills training, job-seeking skills, and job interviewing. The client's psychosocial aspects of adolescent development, such as problems of separation, independence, body image, sexual identity, on-job social skills, and aggression, have not been addressed. Thus, rehabilitation programs for the disabled adolescent may fail in maintenance, because they concentrate exclusively on the specifics of vocational training and not on psychosocial aspects of securing and maintaining employment. Furthermore, although the majority of public school programs provide in-school work experience and summer work programs, these programs are characterized as lacking in the development of requisite social skills.

ADOLESCENT DEVELOPMENTAL TASKS

Research and clinical experience show that the adolescent with developmental disabilities must be helped to resolve the developmental tasks of adolescence before entering vocational training programs (Goldberg, 1981). A comprehensive approach therefore is indicated which responds not only to vocational aspects but also to the preparation of the adolescent in psychosocial aspects for the labor force. For the developmentally disabled adolescent, dysfunctional behavior results from faulty interactions within or across systems involving the individual, family, school, occupation, and community (Davidson & Rappoport, 1983; Szymula & Schleser, 1986). Successful employment therefore hinges upon an ecological approach where responsibility is shared among the individual, his/her employers, educational institutions, and rehabilitation facilities (Rochlin, DeCaro, & Clarcq, 1985). This approach recognizes the importance of the individual's characteristics, the characteristics of the environment, and their interactions (Rusch, 1986). Improving the "communicative interactions" of disabled individuals and significant others (co-workers, employer, etc.) within their ecological systems is the key to their successful non-sheltered employment, because communication is the essence of relationships and relationships are the primary ingredients of supportive employment environments (Rubin, 1983).

Although never easy for the able-bodied youth, the tasks of adolescence, when superimposed upon the burdens caused by chronic physical or mental disability, are laden particularly by conflict and strife. Any rehabilitation program established for the disabled adolescent must first attend to the resolution of normative developmental tasks including separation, body image, sexual identity, and independence (Goldberg, 1981).

Separation

For the disabled adolescent, prolonged medical treatment and chronic institutionalization or hospitalization intensify the conflict of separation. The problems of separation are even greater when the adolescent has substantial psychosocial stress. "Caretaker overprotection" can interfere with successful separation. For example, parents and other caretakers often do not feel vocational success is a realistic goal for the severely developmentally disabled and may refuse to believe and support rehabilitation personnel. Adolescents with developmental disabilities consequently may be caught in a conflict between caretakers who feel too much is being expected of them and rehabilitation personnel who feel too little is expected of them (Bernstein & Karan, 1979).

Body Image

For adolescents with developmental disabilities with obvious physical handicaps, such as paraplegia, spina bifida, and muscular dystrophy, the problem of incorporating a distorted body image into the self-concept becomes crucial (Goldberg, 1981). There is the necessity for a change in employment values so that the personal assets of the disabled individual may be substituted for a comparative value based on physical appearance. Moreover, cognitive interventions may be necessary to facilitate a more adequate self-concept.

Sexual Identity

The adolescent with developmental disabilities has special problems in resolving the developmental task of sexual identity (Schinke, 1984). In a recent study of 430 developmentally disabled adolescents exposed to a sex education program, it was found that many students showed positive changes toward their sexual feeling and were more open about communicating their feelings. In another study of adolescents with learning disabilities, consisting of a heterogeneous group of young men and women (ages 16 to 22) with cognitive and behavioral problems, students' responses to sex education workshops varied from acceptance to anxiety. Adolescents with sensory disabilities have particular difficulty in learning sexual roles and functions (Goldberg, 1981). Lack of crucial interpersonal skills has been implicated in incidence of unwanted sexual intercourse and inconsistent or non-use of contraception (Gilchrist, 1981).

Achieving Independence

The adolescent with developmental disabilities has difficulty in achieving emotional and financial independence. Society has encouraged the child with developmental disabilities, characterized by marked dependence upon parents, friends, and health professionals for the treatment and care of the disability, to remain dependent in sheltered situations at home and school (Goldberg, 1981). The pattern of learned helplessness may hinder the adolescent with developmental disabilities from taking those steps required to prepare for independent living in the community. To achieve independence, data suggest adolescents should be taught the following requisite skills:

1. Personal care—hygiene and care of clothing;
2. Social skills—etiquette and communication;
3. Domestic living skills—household, food preparation, health awareness; and
4. Budgeting skills—personal income, household finances, consumer skills.

Anger Control

During the adolescent years, the aggressive drive is reinforced by changes in the endocrine system and accelerated physical development. However, the capacity to control the aggressive drive is greatly limited during adolescence. Rehabilitation programs may be offered the adolescent to help resolve problems in a socially acceptable way and to adjust the person's aggression to the needs of society (Goldberg, 1981).

SOCIAL BEHAVIORS ASSOCIATED WITH JOB LOSS

The social reasons for job loss fall into three categories: (1) character or moral reasons (e.g. assaulting others, sporadic work attendance); (2) temperament or affective reasons (e.g. yelling, banging head, hallucinations); and (3) social awareness, not understanding people and work settings (e.g. walking into a meeting and talking about a TV program, being inquisitive about other people's business) (Greenspan & Shoultz, 1981). Of the three categories, social awareness incompetence accounted for more job losses than either character or temperament. The ability to understand what other people think and feel, to solve social problems, and to interpret social rules, situations and norms are important behaviors that adolescents with developmental disabilities need to secure and maintain employment.

Kochany and Keller (1981) found that the majority of handicapped individuals lost their jobs for social incompetence (e.g. complaining, screaming, destroying property, interacting inappropriately with supervisors and co-workers, displaying stereotypical and self-abusive behaviors, and being non-compliant). Secondly, several individuals were fired for being excessively tardy or for poor attendance. A third category used to classify reasons for job termination, critical non-vocational reasons, included the social behaviors of poor communication and conversation ability.

The social reasons for job loss reported by other investigators included non-compliance, failure to notify an employer when unable to report for work, and bizarre and aggressive behavior (Wehman, Hill, Goodall, Cleveland, & Pentecost, 1982). Relations with peers and supervisors, inappropriate behaviors, absenteeism and tardiness, poor motivation and attitude, hypochondria, gross insubordination and abusive behavior, and refusal to accept instructions were reported to lead to job loss by Brickey, Campbell, and Browning (1985).

In summary, lack of social skills accounts for 42 percent of all job losses among persons with disabilities. In particular, poor social interactions with employers and co-workers (12%), emotional outbursts (6%), and inappropriate language (3%) contributed to job terminations (Ford, Dineer, & Hall, 1984).

EMPLOYMENT PREQUISITES

A job preparation program's main focus is to prepare handicapped clients for employment by providing training and preparation in the skills and behaviors that constitute employability and by arranging for appropriate job placement. Employability refers to the skills, attitudes, and work behaviors that are necessary to obtain a job and to perform satisfactorily. Placeability refers to the perceived attractiveness of an applicant to an employer. Labor market conditions and an employer's willingness to hire a person with a disability affect a client's placeability.

The most comprehensive operational definitions of employability and placeability are provided by the 339 behaviors assessed by the Vocational Behavior Checklist (VBC; Walls, Zane, & Werner, 1978) which cover seven areas of employment-related competence. As Bolton (1981) stated:

(1) Pre-vocational skills include knowledge about the need for work, what a job is, and the trainee's own vocational interest (e.g., folding, sorting, and the like).

(2) Job related skills refer to the skills that each worker must have to "get around," locate particular characteristics of the work setting.

(3) Work performance skills include such behaviors as setting up the

work station, starting work on time, following instructions and models, sorting and using materials, using and caring for tools, working safely, seeking help, etc.

(4) On-the-job social skills include being friendly to others, following accepted communication procedures, being able to deal constructively with criticism, refraining from socially destructive or annoying behaviors, talking, answering, and touching others appropriately, etc.

(5) Union-financial security skills are concerned with economic considerations, such as obtaining pay, overtime, union functions, budgeting, etc.

(6) Job seeking skills refer to those behaviors involved in locating and applying for employment, such as matching skills with jobs, completing applications, preparing a resume, etc.

(7) Interview skills are the behaviors involved in preparing to be interviewed and in presenting a favorable and accurate impression of self in a job interview. (Pp. 40–41.)

A CONCEPTUAL MODEL FOR EMPLOYMENT

To secure and maintain employment, adolescents with developmental disabilities must exhibit behaviors that are valued and considered appropriate in employment settings. Two major behavioral categories for ensuring employment success include "production skills" and "effective social skills."

Social Skills Training

The comprehensive employment preparation approach is based on an amalgamation of Goldstein and his colleagues' (1980) structured learning model, "Skillstreaming the Adolescent"; Gazda's (1982) life span development skills training approach; Schinke and Gilchrist's (1984) life skills counseling with adolescents program; and Gurney's (1977) relationship enhancement model. The emphasis is on imparting transferable work skills-attitudes rather than training for either specific vocational skills or basic skills such as reading and mathematics. There is "very little evidence to support the proposition that employers are handicapped by the fact that employees lack the basic skills" (Rodriguez, 1980, p. 26). Furthermore, vocational training teaches skills specific to one job; and frequently in today's rapidly expanding technology, these skills become quickly antiquated. Developmentally disabled youths need life management skills which are transferable from one job to the next and from work to home (Dayton, 1978; Dew, 1983). However, skills training per se is not enough. To enable high-risk youths to cope with present stresses and to facilitate their adolescent development, individual and group counseling are essential (Shore, 1977; Zalinger, 1969).

Social skills may be thought of as overt (verbal and non-verbal components of overt social behaviors) and covert (internal skills affecting self-control and problem-solving abilities across all social settings and circumstances) learned behaviors that maximize chances for obtaining positive reinforcement from social interactions while minimizing cost to self and others (Gilchrist, 1981).

Social skills training typically consists of the following components: (1) a rationale as to why a given social behavior is desirable, (2) an opportunity to observe examples of the behavior (i.e. modeling), (3) an opportunity to practice the behavior, usually in role-play situations, and (4) corrective feedback regarding performance (Rusch, 1986).

Research indicates that it is necessary to teach youths with developmental disabilities the work skills and attitudes necessary for them to successfully compete in the job market; handle current problems and stresses; anticipate and prevent future problems; and advance their mental health, social functioning and economic welfare. Initially, adolescents' vocational aptitude and work skills-attitudes should be assessed. Subsequently, they should participate in a series of psychoeducational "courses," including vocational enrichment (Azrin, 1978); enhancing interpersonal relationships (Lange & Jakubowski, 1976); managing stress and building social responsibility (Schinke & Gilchrist, 1984); determining alternatives to aggression and dealing with feelings (Goldstein, Sprafkin, Gershaw, & Klein, 1980); and problem-solving (D'Zurilla & Goldfried, 1971; Spivack & Shure, 1974).

A variety of psychoeducational methods are employed in the "courses," including individual and group counseling, self-assessments, live and videotape demonstrations, behavioral rehearsal with counselor, peer and videotape feedback, written materials, positive reinforcement, individual and group contracts, buddy systems, and progress logs. Most of these therapeutic strategies are delivered through a group work approach (Feldman & Wodarski, 1975; Wodarski, 1981).

THE GROUP CONTEXT FOR TRAINING

Even though recent years have witnessed a growing emphasis on group treatment, relatively few developmentally disabled youth are treated in this manner. The provision of services in groups offers the following positive aspects. The group interactional situation more frequently typifies many kinds of daily interactions. Services that facilitate the development of behaviors which enable people to interact in groups are likely to better prepare them for participation in larger society; that is, will help them learn social skills necessary to secure reinforcement (Feldman & Wodarski, 1975; Wodarski, 1981). From a social learning theory perspective, it is posited that if an employment preparation behavior is learned in a group context, it is likely to come under the control of a greater number of discriminative stimuli; therefore, greater generalization of the behavior can occur for a broader variety of interactional contexts including the work environment.

The group context of the comprehensive employment preparation program is intended to capitalize on the adolescent's dependence on peers. Group identity and cohesion should be fostered within groups of adolescents. Group support can be mobilized to aid individuals at moments of particular difficulty (Ross & Glaser, 1973). The group interaction situation typifies many kinds of daily living situations, and the group provides a context where new behaviors can be tested in a realistic atmosphere (Feldman & Wodarski, 1975).

There are additional substantiated rationales for working with individuals in groups. Groups provide a context where new behaviors can be tested in a realistic atmosphere. Adolescents can get immediate peer feedback and support regarding their problem-solving behaviors. They are provided with role models to facilitate the acquisition of requisite social behavior. Groups provide a more valid locus for accurate diagnosis and a more potent means for changing client behavior (Meyer & Smith, 1977; Rose, 1977; Wodarski, 1981).

Lack of interpersonal relationship skills plays a significant role in the developmentally disabled youth's inability to secure and maintain employment and in their general dissatisfaction with life. Services structured in a group manner should help these individuals practice necessary social skills to facilitate their acquisition, thus enhancing their interpersonal relationships and employment opportunities. Additionally, many developmentally disabled youth feel emptiness, social isolation and a sense of failure and could benefit from the support derived from the group. Finally, the provision of services through groups greatly increases the number of clients who can be served by an effective treatment program (Wodarski & Bagarozzi, 1979).

SPECIFIC ELEMENTS OF THE EMPLOYMENT PARADIGM

The Comprehensive Employment Preparation (CEP) Program occurs three months prior to employment and continues three months after the youth is in the community. This plan bridges the transition between pre-employment and the community workplace.

Programs to accomplish the acquisition of requisite skills in each of the general target areas are chosen from the technology of applied behavioral analysis and social psychology. Recent reviews of problem-solving training programs (D'Zurilla & Goldfried, 1971; Goldfried & Goldfried, 1975; Spivack & Shure, 1974) and cognitive anger control and interpersonal skills training (Lange & Jakubowski, 1976; Rich & Schroeder, 1976; Schinke & Rose, 1976; Wodarski & Hedrick, 1987) have shown that their effectiveness is substantial as compared to other treatment programs for the acquisition of such behaviors. Data supporting vocational enrichment programs from this applied perspective also are impressive (Azrin, 1978; Azrin, Flores, & Kaplan, 1975; Jones & Azrin, 1973). Following are brief descriptions of the program components.

Vocational Achievement Enrichment Program: Pursuing a Job

The vocational enrichment program is based on the work of Azrin (1978), Azrin, Flores, and Kaplan (1975), and Jones and Azrin (1973). General components to be emphasized are:

(1) Group discussions involving strong motivation for vocational achievement. These discussions involve mutual assistance among job seekers, development of a supportive buddy system, family support, sharing of job leads, and widening the variety of positions considered.

(2) Employment-securing aids such as searching want ads, role playing interview situations, instructions in telephoning for appointments, procedures for motivating the job seeker, developing appropriate conversational competencies, emphasizing strong personal attributes in terms of dress and grooming, and securing transportation for job interviews.

(3) Specific things that will be addressed are the counselor's role, how to operate the job club, initial contact with prospective employers, finding employment leads, arranging interviews and analogous

activities, applying for the job, completing the application, simulating the job interview, learning how to answer questions, presenting strong points, learning how to ask appropriate questions, securing and maintaining the job in terms of interpersonal skills, and dealing with rejection.

Rationale. Data indicate that youth with developmental disabilities who have work or work possibilities can become more independent (Shafer, 1987).

Cognitive Anger Control

It has been estimated that approximately 30 percent of developmentally disabled youth lack means to control anger (Benson, Rice, & Miranti, 1986; LeCroy, 1983; May, 1986). Professionals must be prepared to help at-risk developmentally disabled adolescents develop the following behaviors:

(1) Identification of stresses which can provoke anger and subsequent violent behavior.
(2) Development of cognitive relaxation skills to reduce the effects of stresses.
(3) Learning how to receive assertions and deal with others' anger.
(4) Development of appropriate communication and assertion skills.
(5) Practicing alternate behavior, such as stimulus removal, in anger-provoking situations.

Rationale. Recent data suggest that within six weeks of employment, developmentally disabled youths have altercations that lead to their termination (Feindler & Ecton, 1986).

Problem Solving

Developmentally disabled youths and young adults who have difficulties maintaining employment are deficient in their ability to cope with the daily problems of living in terms of personal care, domestic living skills, and budgeting skills (Agran & Martin, 1987). These youths can be taught a problem-solving approach based on the work of D'Zurilla and Goldfried (1971), Goldfried and Goldfried (1975), Schinke and Gilchrist (1984), and Spivack and Shure (1974). The general components emphasized are:

(1) How to generate information
(2) How to generate possible solutions

(3) How to evaluate possible courses of action
(4) Ability to choose and implement strategies through the following procedures:
    (a) general introduction to how the provision of certain consequences and stimuli can control problem-solving behavior
    (b) isolation and definition of a behavior to be changed
    (c) use of stimulus control techniques to influence rates of problem-solving behavior
    (d) use of appropriate consequences to either increase or decrease a behavior
(5) Verification of the outcome of the chosen course of action

Rationale. Data indicate that from an early age institutionalized developmentally disabled youth and young adults do not solve problems as readily as other individuals (Farley, 1984; Stark & Kiernan, 1986).

The Social Skills Program

This component is based on the work of Lange and Jakubowski (1976) and involves interpersonal skills training and the development of assertive behavior for appropriate situations. Specific elements emphasized include:

(1) How to introduce oneself
(2) How to initiate conversations and continue them
(3) Giving and receiving compliments
(4) Enhancing appearance
(5) Making and refusing requests
(6) Spontaneous expression of feelings
(7) Appropriate use of non-verbal distance, body language, face, hand and foot movement, and smiling
(8) Appropriate sexuality

Rationale. Data indicate that from an early age developmentally disabled youth are disliked by their peers and do not possess the interpersonal skills necessary to interact well with others (Hill, Wehman, Hill, & Goodall, 1986; Roessler & Lewis, 1984).

DISCUSSION

To secure and maintain employment it is necessary to help youth and young adults with developmental disabilities acquire socially sanctioned skills which lead to procurement of employment and to train them to interact in appropriate ways with their peers and employers on the job.

Although numerous projects have been conducted to help young people with developmental disabilities deal with employment problems, few have approached the problem in a comprehensive manner. Programs should not only facilitate adolescents' orientation to work but must also provide them with skills and attitudes for healthy living. Although previous programs have used a combination of counseling, education and work to assist developmentally disabled youth, none have combined the recent development in social skills training as this comprehensive program proposes to do. The program of youth employment, especially for developmentally disabled youth, will remain with us in the foreseeable future. Ideally, emphasis will be on prevention rather than remediation of job-related problems through job preparation programs of the nature described here.

The Comprehensive Employment Preparation Program offers an exciting and functional method of equipping youth and young adults with developmental disabilities to become productive members of society by building alternative positive behaviors that have a higher probability of reducing dependence. The available data indicate that this is the best avenue worth pursuing. The benefits of the approach are substantial. It is based on available data to indicate what works; the approach is less costly than those approaches currently in use; and in today's employment-conscious society, the program will most likely be supported by the general public.

FUTURE RESEARCH ISSUES

A number of research issues remain to be addressed in the future. First, even though social behaviors are important in job situations, little agreement has been reached regarding how to define, measure, assess, and teach social skills. Moreover, it must be determined which of the numerous behaviors are the most relevant.

Second, little is known about the important social tasks that involve interacting with others that exist in employment settings. Social tasks must be identified and adequately described. Furthermore, tasks must be described in relation to specific jobs, generalities across jobs, and variables (e.g setting, criteria) that may affect them. For example, "washing dishes," "sweeping the floor," and "carrying out the garbage" are production-related tasks that exist in employment settings. Research must isolate the relevant corresponding social behaviors (Rusch, 1986).

Third, supervisors and co-workers play an essential role in the development of social competence of employees with developmental disabilities. How can co-workers and supervisors be more effectively used in training situations? For example, the attitudes (e.g. emotional support, positive reinforcement and setting structure) of co-workers toward disabled individuals can be a good supportive means to develop the social competence of employees with developmental disabilities.

Fourth, parent-professional partnerships may be viewed as one of the most critical elements in a vocational training program, because the family exerts a powerful influence on the career attitude and options of the individuals with disabilities. For example, over 80 percent of former special education students who were working obtained employment through a self-family-friend network (Schutz, 1986). Involvement of families in facilitating securing and maintaining employment, however, has been minimal.

Finally, research indicates that teaching self-control procedures to adolescents with mild to moderate developmental disabilities will be a valuable adjunct to successful employment. The actual combination of external (e.g. parents, employers, visual aids, and so forth) and internal (self-thoughts, self-talk, and so forth) cues needs to be isolated (Agran & Martin, 1987).

Relationships among rehabilitation agencies, educational institutions, a person with disabilities, and employers must be developed before, during and after the person is employed by a corporation. Support systems are critical to the attainment and maintenance of employment. Acquisition of entry-level jobs should not be considered the end result of the education and rehabilitation process but rather the commencement of a career.

SUMMARY

This chapter presented a comprehensive employment preparation intervention for adolescents with developmental disabilities. Vocational preparation was viewed in terms of the development of job skills and related psychosocial skills.

The Comprehensive Employment Preparation Program is designed as a means of helping youth and young adults with developmental disabilities acquire skills necessary to prepare them for effective functioning as self-sustaining, *working* members of society. Substantial research indicates that the lack of social, problem-solving and employment-seeking skills is a significant factor in attaining and maintaining employment. At this time, relevant educational and psychological literature clearly reveals progress is being made in our ability to appropriately assess individual deficiencies and program for development of improved social competency, i.e. problem-solving, interpersonal and vocational competencies. Lastly, future policy and research issues were briefly reviewed.

REFERENCES

Agran, M., & Martin, J. E. (1987). Applying a technology of self-control in community environments for individuals who are mentally retarded. In M. Hersen, R. Eisler, & P. Miller (Eds.), *Progress in behavior modification* (Vol. 21, pp. 108-151). Newbury Park: SAGE Publications.

Azrin, N. H. (1978, November). *A learning approach to job finding.* Paper presented at the Association for Advancement of Behavior Therapy, Chicago.

Azrin, H. H., Flores, T., & Kaplan, S. J. (1975). Job-finding club: A group program for obtaining employment. *Behavior Research and Therapy, 13,* 17-27.

Benson, B. A., Rice, C. J., & Miranti, S. V. (1986). Effects of anger management training with mentally retarded adults in group treatment. *Journal of Consulting and Clinical Psychology, 54*(5), 728-729.

Bernstein, G. S., & Karan, O. C. (1979, March). Obstacles to vocational normalization for the developmentally disabled. *Rehabilitation Literature,* 66-71.

Bolton, B. (1981). Assessing employability of handicapped persons: The vocational rehabilitation perspective. *Journal of Applied Rehabilitation Counseling, 12*(1), 40-44.

Briar, K. H. (1976). *The effect of long-term unemployment on workers and their families.* DSW dissertation, The University of California at Berkeley.

Brickey, M. P., Campbell, K. M., & Browning, L. J. (1985). A five-year follow-up of sheltered workshop employees placed in competitive jobs. *Mental Retardation, 23,* 67-83.

Canonico, A., & Lombardi, T. P. (1984). Effects of career adaptive behavior activities in mentally handicapped students. *Exceptional Children, 50*(6), 545-546.

Coles, R. (1976). Work and self-respect. *Daedalus, 105*(4), 29-38.

Coughran, L., & Daniels, J. L. (1983, January/February/March). Early vocational intervention for the severely handicapped. *Journal of Rehabilitation,* 37-41.

Davidson, W., & Rappoport, J. (1983). Advocacy and community psychology. In G. Weber & G. McCall (Eds.), *Social scientists as advocates.* Beverly Hills: SAGE.

Dayton, C. W. (1978, March). The dimensions of youth unemployment. *Journal of Employment Counseling,* 3-27.

Dayton, C. W. (1981). The young person's job search: Insights from a study. *Journal of Counseling Psychology, 28,* 321-333.

Dew, A. (1983). Personal communication. University of Alabama at Birmingham, July 1.

D'Zurilla, T. J., & Goldfried, M. R. (1971). Problem solving and behavior modification. *Journal of Abnormal Psychology, 78,* 101-126.

Farley, R. C. (1984, December). Training in rational-behavior problem solving and employability enhancement of rehabilitation clients. *Rehabilitation Counseling Bulletin,* 117-123.

Feindler, E. L., & Ecton, R. B. (1986). *Adolescent anger control: Cognitive-behavioral techniques.* Elmsford, NY: Pergamon.

Feldman, R. A., & Wodarski, J. S. (1975). *Contemporary approaches to group treatment.* San Francisco: Jossey-Bass.

Ferguson, D. L., & Ferguson, P. M. (1986). The new victors: A progressive policy analysis of work reform for people with very severe handicaps. *Mental Retardation, 24*(6), 331-338.

Ford, L., Dineer, J., & Hall, J. (1984). Is there life after placement? *Education & Training of the Mentally Retarded, 19,* 291-296.

Gallup Organization. (1980). *American families, 1980: A summary of findings.* Princeton, NJ.

Gazda, G. M. (1982). Life skills training. In E. Marshall & D. Kurtz (Eds.), *Interpersonal helping skills.* San Francisco: Jossey-Bass.

Gilchrist, L. D. (1981). Social competence in adolescence. In S. Schinke (Ed.), *Behavioral methods in social-welfare* (pp. 61-80). New York: Aldine.

Goldberg, R. T. (1981, March/April). Toward an understanding of the rehabilitation of the disabled adolescent. *Rehabilitation Literature,* 66-73.

Goldfried, M., & Goldfried, A. (1975). Cognitive change methods. In F. Kanfer & A. Goldstein (Eds.), *Helping people change.* New York: Pergamon.

Goldstein, A. P., Sprafkin, R. P., Gershaw, N. J., & Klein, P. (1980). *Skillstreaming the adolescent.* Champaign, IL: Research Press.

Greenberger, E., & Steinberg, L. (1986). *When teenagers work: The psychological and social costs of adolescent employment.* New York: Basic Books, Inc.

Greenspan, S., & Shoultz, B. (1981). Why mentally retarded adults lost their jobs: Social incompetence as a factor in work adjustment. *Applied Research in Mental Retardation, 2,* 23-38.

Gurney, B. G. (1977). *Relationship enhancement.* San Francisco: Jossey-Bass.

Hill, J. W., Wehman, P., Hill, M., & Goodall, P. (1986). Differential reasons for job separation of previously employed persons with mental retardation. *Mental Retardation, 24*(6), 347-352.

Jones, J., & Azrin, N. H. (1973). An experimental application of a social reinforcement approach to the problem of job finding. *Journal of Applied Behavior Analysis, 6,* 345-353.

Karan, O. C., & Knight, C. B. (1983). Developing support networks for individuals who fail to achieve competitive employment. In F. Rusch (Ed.), *Competitive employment issues and strategies* (pp. 241-255). Baltimore: Paul H. Brookes.

Kochany, L., & Keller, J. (1981). An analysis and evaluation of the failures of severely disabled individuals in competitive employment. In P. Wehman (Ed.),

Competitive employment: New horizons for severely disabled individuals (pp. 181-198). Baltimore: Paul H. Brookes.

Lange, A. J., & Jakubowski, P. (1976). *Responsible assertive behavior.* Champaign, IL: Research Press.

LeCroy, C. W. (1983). Social-cognitive group work with children. *Behavior Group Therapy, 5*(1), 9-12.

May, J. M. (1986). Cognitive processes and violent behavior in young people. *Journal of Adolescence, 9,* 17-27.

Meyer, R. G., & Smith, S. S. (1977). A crisis in group therapy. *American Psychologist, 32,* 638-643.

Rich, A. H., & Schroeder, H. E. (1976). Research issues in assertiveness training. *Psychological Bulletin, 83,* 1081-1096.

Riggar, T. F. (1979, October). Stages in the rehabilitation of the developmental disabled. *Rehabilitation Literature,* 305-308.

Rochlin, J. F., DeCaro, J. J., & Clarcq, J. R. (1985, April/May/June). Competitive employment of disabled people: The need for a partnership. *Journal of Rehabilitation,* 19-23.

Rodriguez, J. F. (1980). Youth employment: A need assessment. In *A review of youth employment problems, programs and policies: The youth employment problem* (Vol. 1). Washington, DC: U. S. Government Printing Office.

Roessler, R. T., & Lewis, F. D. (1984, January). Conversation skill training with mentally retarded and learning disabled sheltered workshop clients. *Rehabilitation Counseling Bulletin,* 161-171.

Rose, S. D. (1977). *Group therapy: A behavioral approach.* Englewood Cliffs, NJ: Prentice-Hall.

Ross, H., & Glaser, E. (1973). Making it out of the ghetto. *Professional Psychology, 4*(3), 347-356.

Rubin, T. I. (1983). *One to one understanding of personal relationships.* New York: Viking Press.

Rusch, F. R. (1986). *Competitive employment issues and strategies.* Baltimore: Paul H. Brookes.

Rusch, J. C. (1986). Identifying and teaching social behaviors. In F. Rusch (Ed.), *Competitive employment issues and strategies* (pp. 273-282). Baltimore: Paul H. Brookes.

Schinke, S. P. (1984). Preventing teenage pregnancy. In M. Hersen et al. (Eds.), *Progress in behavior modification* (Vol. 16, pp. 31-64). Orlando: Academic.

Schinke, S. P., & Gilchrist, L. D. (1984). *Life skills counseling with adolescents.* Baltimore: University Park Press.

Schinke, S. P., & Rose, S. D. (1976). Interpersonal skill training in groups. *Journal of Counseling Psychology, 23,* 442-448.

Schutz, R. P. (1986). Establishing a parent-professional partnership to facilitate competitive employment. In F. Rusch (Ed.), *Competitive employment issues and strategies* (pp. 289-302). Baltimore: Paul H. Brookes.

Shafer, M. S. (1987). Competitive employment for workers with mental retardation. In M. Hersen, R. Eisler, & P. Miller (Eds.), *Progress in behavior modification* (Vol. 21, pp. 86-107). Newbury Park, CA: SAGE.

Shore, M. R. (1977). Evaluation of a community-based clinical program for antisocial youth. *Evaluation, 4,* 104-107.

Spivack, G., & Shure, M. B. (1974). *Social adjustment of young children.* San Francisco: Jossey-Bass.

Stark, J. A., & Kiernan, W. E. (1986). Symposium overview: Employment for people with mental retardation. *Mental Retardation, 24*(6), 329-330.

Szymula, G., & Schleser, R. C. (1986). A reappraisal of vocational education from an ecological systems perspective. *Rehabilitation Literature, 47*(9-10), 224-228.

U. S. Commission on Civil Rights. (1983, September). *Accommodating the spectrum of disabilities.* Washington, DC: U. S. Commission on Civil Rights.

Walls, R. T., Zane, T., & Werner, T. J. (1978). *The vocational behavior checklist* (expanded edition). Morgantown: West Virginia Rehabilitation Research & Training Center.

Wehman, P., Hill, M., Goodall, P., Cleveland, V. B., & Pentecost, J. (1982). Job placements and follow-up of moderately and severely handicapped individuals after three years. *Journal of the Association for Severely Handicapped, 7,* 5-15.

Wehman, P., Kregel, J., & Zoller, K. (1984). *A follow-up of mentally retarded graduates' vocational and independent living skills in Virginia.* Manuscript in preparation.

Wodarski, J. S. (1981). *Role of research in clinical practice.* Austin, TX: PRO-ED.

Wodarski, J. S., & Hedrick, M. (1987). Violent children: A practice paradigm. *Social Work in Education, 10*(1), 28-42.

Wodarski, J. S., & Bagarozzi, D. A. (1979). *Behavioral social work.* New York: Human Sciences Press.

Zalinger, A. D. (1969). Job training programs: Motivational and structural dimensions. *Poverty and Human Abstracts, 4*(3), 5-13.

Chapter 9

FAMILY INTERVENTION

DATA INDICATE THAT parents whose adolescents are at risk face multiple social and psychological difficulties. The clearest empirical finding with regard to adolescents at risk seems to be the lack of consistency by the parent or parents in the handling of their children and the consequent lack of effectiveness in managing the child's behavior in a manner that facilitates their psychological and social development. It has also been pointed out that another common feature of relationships between parents and adolescents at risk is unrealistic expectations by the parents regarding what is appropriate behavior for their child (Patterson & Forgatch, 1987; Wodarski & Thyer, in press).

Another empirical finding of substance has been the high degree of strain evident in families. Family interaction patterns have been characterized as primarily negative; that is, parents engage in excessive amounts of criticism, threats, negative statements, physical punishment, and a corresponding lack of positive interaction such as positive statements, praise, positive physical contact, and so forth (Bock & English, 1973; Brandon & Folk, 1977; Brennan, Huizinga, & Elliott, 1978; Hildebrand, 1968; Robinson, 1978; Suddick, 1973; Vandeloo, 1977). In view of this finding, a comprehensive prevention approach should include appropriate interventions that teach knowledge about the problems adolescents face, communication skills, problem solving, and conflict resolution to family members.

EMPHASIS ON CHILD MANAGEMENT TRAINING AND BEHAVIORAL TECHNIQUES IN THE PREVENTION OF ADOLESCENT MALTREATMENT

There have been numerous studies linking behavior management techniques to treatment and prevention of adolescent maltreatment.

Identification of specific, observable problem behaviors is essential, as well as identification of specific coping skills for parents (Belsky, 1970). Parents can learn what to expect in terms of behaviors from adolescents at different stages of life. They learn to consistently reward adolescents for good behaviors and to use stimulus control to alter adolescents' misbehaviors (Mastria, Mastria, & Hawkins, 1979; Polkov & Peabody, 1975; Resnick & Sweet, 1979; Tracy & Clark, 1974; Wodarski & Bagarozzi, 1979). Contingency contracting, discrimination training, and assertiveness training are all parts of such a preventive approach. Time-out procedures frequently are used (Polkov & Peabody, 1975). Keeping charts of observable behaviors has been determined to be quite a successful practice in preventing misbehaviors by parents and adolescents (Tracy & Clark, 1974). Modeling of appropriate behaviors by an instructor in class is important to demonstrate acceptable role models (Belsky, 1970). Behaviors are broken into small, achievable steps. Videotaped sessions of interactions between parent and adolescent have been used successfully in prevention programs (Mastria et al., 1979). Classes emphasizing reinforcement of anger control have also been used in conjunction with preventing adolescent maltreatment (Resnick & Sweet, 1979). Such classes have focused on role playing, listening skills, and even homework assignments for parents (Rinn & Markle, 1977). Special attention has been focused toward improving the consistency of parenting skills, as that factor seems to be linked to adolescent maltreatment (Resnick & Sweet, 1979). Paul S. Graubard in his book, *Positive Parenthood,* emphasizes the importance of parents' recognizing and reinforcing their adolescents' strengths more than their drawbacks or weaknesses (Graubard, 1977). In fact, a special training procedure has been developed by Doctor Thomas Gordon (1970) of behavior management techniques for parents. In his book, *Parent Effectiveness Training,* Doctor Gordon outlines a specific course (usually eight weekly sessions, each 3 hours long) for target parents. The course covers parent-child communication, guidelines for listening skills, and a no-lose method for solving conflicts (Gordon, 1970). The behavior management approach may be appealing and successful, because it focuses on what to teach and tells one how (Graubard, 1977).

What are some of the general and specific advantages to behavioral approaches? Gelfand and Hartman (1968) state that there are several advantages to behavioral management classes. These include: that the practices are empirically based; the number of individuals dealt with at one time is large; the training period is relatively short-term in nature;

the training requires a small professional staff; the training is not based on a sickness model; and lastly, a large percentage of adolescent problems can be broken into specific behaviors suitable for change by this training (O'Dell, 1974).

Why should such training be appropriate? There are numerous reasons. Perhaps the most important concerns the language used. Behavior management can be presented in easily understandable, frequently observable terms. People of average intelligence and below average education can understand the basic concepts. Parents need terms and procedures that they can easily grasp, that they can relate to, and that are relevant to their everyday lives. They do not need to be bothered with fancy therapy techniques. Likewise, a majority of people could not understand the fancy terminology used in psychotherapy or Gestalt therapy.

Next, the classes break problems and behaviors into small, observable, countable steps. In other words, easy success for parent and adolescent is the key feature of this program. This increases participation and motivation as well as understanding. The programs are relatively short in duration and can serve several families at once, which reduces the cost and increases the served population. Moreover, the classes should be held at night for working parents. Parents can share feelings, interact with and observe role models of other parents, and are likely to benefit from the support derived from being in a group. A skilled leader of such classes does not have to be highly trained or highly paid. He or she can be someone from the community and a successful parent as well. No special equipment is needed to teach these skills. Finally, and of utmost importance, such a program provides a positive approach. It involves no burden of guilt for parents. In fact, classes are very beneficial to all parents because no "sick" label is attached to participants. This encourages participation, dedication, and communication about such a program in a positive, proud way. Behavior management represents the new look of adolescent maltreatment prevention.

Rationale

Behavioral approaches form the major body of the well-controlled, methodologically sound outcome experiments in marital and family intervention. For marital intervention, over 20 rigorous outcome studies document the efficacy of behavioral methods (Baucom, 1987), while over 100 controlled group outcome studies illustrate the value of behavioral methods to improve parent-child relationships, a major focus of family intervention (Dangel & Polster, 1984; Kazdin, 1987).

One simple rationale for training significant others in prevention procedures is the amount of time they spend with each other (Berkowitz & Graziano, 1972; Graziano, 1977; O'Dell, 1974). Moreover, significant others can be trained easily to use contingency management techniques to influence behavior of other family members and to provide appropriate consequences for desired behavior. With proper training, significant others can be taught to identify reinforcers to facilitate the acquisition and maintenance of appropriate behavior, how to use contingency contracting, how to change their own behavior, and so forth. In all of these instances where the training of significant others is involved, once the behavioral procedures are mastered it is essential that significant others apply them consistently (Wodarski, 1987). Families may need behavioral intervention to increase reciprocity and positive reinforcement among family members, to establish clear communication, to help specify behavior that family members desire from each other, and to negotiate constructively and help identify solutions to interpersonal difficulties (Wodarski & Thyer, in press).

INTERVENTIONS WITH CHILDREN AND ADOLESCENTS

Once a relationship is strengthened, an impressive body of empirical research describes effective methods to alter child and adolescent behaviors. Each application program described below is supported by numerous credible scientific studies. If the relationship is not strengthened, parents may not provide the consistency in applying continuity of reinforcement to alter the child's behavior; thus, interventions may prove ineffective (Dadds, Schwartz, & Sanders, 1987; Griest & Wells, 1983).

Child Management Program

The child management program rests on one of the impressive data bases in the literature and is based on Patterson's (1971, 1975, 1986), Patterson and Fleischman's (1979), and Jensen's (1976) work with families. The general components that are emphasized include:

(1) General introduction to the behaviors that are appropriate for children at different developmental stages. For example, initial

language skills, ability to identify objects, ability to carry out requests, and so forth.

(2) General introduction to how the provision of certain consequences in terms of rewards and punishments can control behavior. For example, verbal praise, eye contact, or verbal reprimands.

(3) How to isolate and define a behavior to be changed, such as throwing of objects, increased sibling interaction, and increased verbalization.

(4) The use of appropriate consequences to either increase or decrease a behavior such as rewards, punishment, time-out, and extinction.

(5) Use of stimulus control techniques to influence rates of behavior, e.g. restructuring physical aspects of the home, or helping parents to see how certain behaviors, such as raising their voices, losing eye contact, praise, facial expressions, and so forth, control behavior.

(6) Use of simple graphs and tables to chart behavioral change and to show parents the effectiveness of the interventions.

INTERVENTION WITH ADOLESCENTS

Our theoretical perspective is anchored within a broad base of social learning theory (Robin & Foster, 1984). From this viewpoint, the adolescent learns appropriate and inappropriate behavior from the context (that is, parents and peers) in which he/she functions through observational learning and reinforcement (Bandura, 1969). That is, by observing the behaviors demonstrated by others and by subsequently receiving or not receiving reinforcement/punishment for engaging in such behaviors, adolescents acquire certain behavior patterns. Moreover, the use of different schedules of reinforcement and punishment by parents and siblings effect the strength of the behavioral patterns to change. Furthermore, and of particular importance, if an adolescent functions within a context in which good communication skills and/or adequate knowledge is lacking [e.g. he/she has inadequate knowledge and unrealistic beliefs, expectations, or attributions (Robin & Foster, 1984)], he/she is more likely to engage in maladaptive behavior patterns through modeling and reinforcement. Such a pathognomonic developmental process may not provide the adolescent with the requisite behaviors for prosocial attachment to family members, peers, and social institutions and is a high-risk factor for subsequent adolescent behavioral difficulties.

One of the critical variables that influence an adolescent's development is the family. The particular types of parenting behavior (lack of positive reinforcement, inconsistent or contradictory patterns of reinforcement and punishment, communication skills, and problem-solving skills) can serve as predictors of adolescent problems (Pulkkinen, 1983) and can discriminate between adolescents at high risk of developing subsequent interpersonal difficulties (Rees & Wilborn, 1983).

Basically, problem solving involves four steps: problem identification, generation of alternative solutions, decision making, and planning solution implementation (Robin & Foster, 1984). Communication involves skills which can be used during problem-solving discussions and at other times. Robin and Foster (1984) have identified 20 behaviors that may interfere with effective communication. These include accusing, putting down, interrupting, getting off topics, dwelling on the past, and threatening, among others. Robin, Foster and their colleagues have conducted three well-controlled studies which support the effectiveness of a problem-solving communication skills training program for parents. Relative to waiting list control groups and a family therapy approach, problem-solving communications skills training increases communication and decreases conflicts (Foster, Prinz, & O'Leary, 1983; Robin, 1981; Robin, Kent, O'Leary, Foster, & Prinz, 1977). Furthermore, at follow-up, improvements achieved with problem-solving skills were maintained. Therefore, it would appear that teaching parents to provide appropriate models and improving parents' problem-solving and communication skills would be critical ingredients of an adolescent intervention program.

Family Interaction Skills Development

In the family intervention component, parents participate in a six-week program in which they meet in groups (both parents, if possible) two hours each week. The initial focus is on development of knowledge about the problems adolescents face and the dynamics of how families function as systems of rewards and punishments. Presentation of the social learning theory aspects of behavioral development and parents' roles in altering and maintaining adolescents' behavior are reviewed. Parents see how to use stimulus control techniques to influence rates of behavior and to provide appropriate consequences for desired behavior. Parents are taught to identify motivators to facilitate the acquisition and maintenance of appropriate behaviors, how to use contingency contracting, how to change their own behavior, and so forth. Parents' roles in maintenance of behavior is stressed. This information is dispensed in handouts and is covered within the first and second two-hour group sessions and, where appropriate, in the other four sessions.

The third and fourth sessions are devoted to teaching problem-solving skills and communication skills for conflict resolution based on Robin and Foster's (1984) work. The five steps involved in problem solving are delineated: problem definition, generation of alternate solutions, decision making, planning solution implementation, and renegotiation. Parents initially are presented with these steps in a rather formal manner. Topics are discussed in the group and then role plays of how to use the procedures are implemented. The role play consists of selected group members attempting to solve problems of adolescents of other group members.

When the basic steps for problem solving have been delineated and practiced, communication training will be implemented. The communication targets (Robin & Foster, 1984) listed in Table 9-1 are distributed to parents. The various problematic behaviors are discussed as well as the possible alternatives. Presentation of problematic and appropriate behavior is conducted by group leaders. Subsequently, various participants role-play problem-solving situations and receive feedback from other group members concerning their use of communication/conflict resolution skills.

Table 9-1

DICTIONARY OF COMMUNICATION TARGETS

Problematic Behavior	*Possible Alternative*
1. Talking through a third person.	Talking directly to another person.
2. Accusing, blaming, defensive statements.	Making I-statements (I feel _____ when _____ happens).
3. Putting down, zapping, shaming.	Accepting responsibility, I-statement.
4. Interrupting (other than for clarification).	Listening; raising hand or gesturing when wanting to talk. Encouraging speakers to use brief statements.
5. Overgeneralizing, catastrophizing, making extremist, rigid statements.	Qualifying, making tentative statements (sometimes, maybe, etc.); accurate quantitative statements.

Table 9-1 *(continued)*

Problematic Behavior	*Possible Alternative*
6. Lecturing, preaching, moralizing	Making brief, explicit problem statements (I would like _____).
7. Talking in a sarcastic tone of voice.	Talking in a neutral tone of voice.
8. Failing to make eye contact.	Looking at the person with whom you are talking.
9. Fidgeting, moving restlessly, or gesturing while being spoken to.	Sitting in a relaxed fashion. Excusing self for being restless.
10. Mindreading (attributing thoughts and feelings to another without the other's having communicated these feelings).	Reflecting, paraphrasing, validating.
11. Getting off the topic.	Catching self and returning to the problem as defined.
12. Commanding, ordering.	Suggesting alternative solutions.
13. Dwelling on the past.	Sticking to the present and future, suggesting changes to correct past problems.
14. Monopolizing the conversation.	Taking turns, making brief statements.
15. Intellectualizing, pedanticizing.	Speaking in simple, clear language that a teenager can understand.
16. Threatening.	Suggesting alternative solutions.
17. Humoring, discounting.	Reflecting, validating.
18. Incongruence between verbal and non-verbal behavior.	Matching verbal affect and non-verbal posture.

In sessions three and four, information is presented on the use of positive and negative control with adolescents. The focus within this material is on increasing use of positive reinforcement for appropriate behavior rather than often used coercive processes such as negative reinforcement and punishment (Forehand & McMahon, 1981; Patterson, 1981).

In the last two sessions, the use of problem-solving, communication training, and positive reinforcement procedures are integrated and applied to resolving adolescent developmental issues. It is emphasized that generally using communication skills, problem-solving skills, and positive reinforcement will result in a better relationship with their adolescents (better communication, less conflict) and, therefore, will reduce the probability of interpersonal difficulties.

SUMMARY

This chapter has elucidated the various paradigms that can be utilized to involve parents to support the acquisition of knowledge and relevant social behaviors in their adolescents. It is emphasized that the procedures need to be concrete and teach specific ways that parents can support their adolescents. Moreover, the delivery of the content should be done in an attractive facilitative manner and usually in six two-hour sessions. A program that does not include the parents in supporting adolescents developing the knowledge and requisite behaviors has a lesser probability of being successful.

REFERENCES

Bandura, A. (1969). *Principles of behavior modification.* New York: Holt, Rinehart, & Winston.

Baucom, D.H. (1987). Marital therapy: A shifting phenomenon. *Contemporary Psychology, 32*(9), 804-805.

Belsky, J. (1970). A theoretical analysis of child abuse remediation strategy. *Journal of Clinical Child Psychology, 7,* 117-120.

Berkowitz, B. P., & Graziano, A. M. (1972). Training parents as behavior therapists: A review. *Behaviour Research and Therapy, 10,* 297-317.

Bock, R., & English, A. (1973). *Got me on the run.* Boston: Beacon.

Brandon, J. S., & Folk, S. (1977). Runaway adolescents' perceptions of parents and self. *Adolescence, 12,* 175-187.

Brennan, T., Huizinga, D., & Elliott, D. S. (1978). *The social psychology of runaways.* Lexington, MA: D. C. Heath.

Dadds, M. R., Schwartz, S., & Sanders, M. R. (1987). Marital discord and treatment outcome in behavioral treatment of child conduct disorders. *Journal of Consulting and Clinical Psychology, 55*(3), 396-403.

Dangel, R. F., & Polster, R. A. (Eds.), (1984). *Parent training: Foundations of research and practice.* New York: Guilford.

Forehand, R. L., & McMahon, R. J. (1981). *Helping the non-compliant child: A clinician's guide to parent training.* New York: Guilford.

Foster, S. L., Prinz, R. J., & O'Leary, K. D. (1983). Impact of problem-solving communication training and generalization procedures on family conflict. *Child and Family Behavior Therapy, 5,* 1-24.

Gelfand, D. M., & Hartman, D. P. (1968). Behavior therapy with children: A review and evaluation of research methodology. *Psychological Bulletin, 69,* 204-215.

Gordon, T. (1970). *Parent effectiveness training.* New York: Plume.

Graubard, P. S. (1977). *Positive parenthood.* New York: Bobbs-Merrill.

Graziano, A. M. (1977). Parents as behavior therapists. In M. Hersen, R. Eisler, & P. Miller (Eds.), *Progress in behavior modification* (Vol. 4). New York: Academic Press.

Griest, D. L., & Wells, K. C. (1983). Behavioral family therapy with conduct disorders in children. *Behavior Therapy, 14*(1), 37-53.

Hildebrand, J. A. (1968). Reasons for runaways. *Crime and Delinquency, 14*(1), 42-48.

Jensen, R. E. (1976). A behavior modification program to remediate child abuse. *Journal of Clinical Child Psychology, 5*(1), 30-32.

Kazdin, A. E. (1987). Treatment of antisocial behavior in children: Current status and future directions. *Psychological Bulletin, 102*(2), 187-203.

Mastria, E. O., Mastria, M., & Hawkins, J. (1979). Treatment of child abuse by behavioral intervention: A case report. *Child Welfare, 58,* 253-263.

O'Dell, S. (1974). Training parents in behavior modification: A review. *Psychological Bulletin, 81,* 418-433.

Patterson, G. R. (1971). *Families: Application of social learning to family life.* Champaign, IL: Research Press.

Patterson, G. R. (1975). *Families.* Eugene, OR: Castalia.

Patterson, G. R. (1981). *Coercive family process.* Eugene, OR: Castalia.

Patterson, G. R. (1986). Performance models for antisocial boys. *American Psychologist, 41,* 432-444.

Patterson, G. R., & Fleischman, M. J. (1979). Maintenance of treatment effects: Some considerations concerning family systems and follow-up data. *Behavior Therapy, 10,* 168-185.

Patterson, G. R., & Forgatch, M. S. (1987). *Parents and adolescents living together. Part 1: The basics.* Eugene, OR: Castalia.

Polkov, R. L., & Peabody, D. (1975). Behavioral treatment for child abusers. *International Journal of Offender Therapy and Comparative Criminology, 19,* 100-102.

Pulkkinen, L. (1983). Youthful smoking and drinking in a longitudinal perspective. *Journal of Youth and Adolescence, 12,* 253-283.

Rees, C. D., & Wilborn, B. L. (1983). Correlates of drug abuse in adolescents: A comparison of families of drug users with families of non-drug users. *Journal of Youth and Adolescence, 12,* 55-63.

Resnick, P., & Sweet, J. J. (1979). The maltreatment of children: A review of theories and research. *Journal of Sociological Issues, 35,* 40-59.

Rinn, R., & Markle, A. (1977). Parent effectiveness training: A review. *Behav Rep, 41,* 95-109.

Robin, A. L. (1981). A controlled evaluation of problem-solving communication training with parent-adolescent conflict. *Behavior Therapy, 12,* 593-609.

Robin, A. L., & Foster, S. L. (1984). Problem-solving communication training: A behavioral family systems approach to parent-adolescent conflict. In P. Karoly & J. Steffen (Eds.), *Adolescent behavior disorders: Foundations and contemporary concerns.* Lexington, MA: Lexington Books.

Robin, A. L., Kent, R., O'Leary, K. D., Foster, S. L., & Prinz, R. (1977). An approach to teaching parents and adolescents problem-solving communication skills: A preliminary report. *Behavior Therapy, 8,* 639-643.

Robinson, P. A. (1978). Parents of "beyond control" adolescents. *Adolescence, 13*(49), 109-119.

Suddick, D. (1973). Runaways: A review of the literature. *Juvenile Justice, 24,* 46-54.

Tracy, J., & Clark, E. (1974). Treatment for child abusers. *Social Work, 19,* 338-342.

Vandeloo, M. C. (1977). A study of coping behavior of runaway adolescents as related to situational stresses. *Dissertation Abstracts International, 38,* 2387-2388B. (University Microfilms No. 5-B)

Wodarski, J. S. (1987). *Social work practice with children and adolescents.* Springfield, IL: Charles C Thomas.

Wodarski, J. S., & Bagarozzi, D. (1979). *Behavioral social work.* New York: Human Sciences Press.

Wodarski, J. S., & Thyer, B. A. (in press). Behavioral perspectives on the family: An overview. In B. Thyer (Ed.), *Behavioral family interventions* (an edited volume in the NCFR/Sage Monograph Series).

Chapter 10

ISSUES IN ADOLESCENT PREVENTION

THESE ARE exciting times in adolescent prevention. A growing body of well-controlled outcome studies now document the effectiveness of a variety of behavioral approaches in improving the behavioral capabilities of at-risk adolescents (Dangel & Polster, 1984; Jacobson & Margolin, 1979; Schinke & Gilchrist, 1984). One may now turn to specific, empirically supported guidelines for intervention with a number of formerly intractable problems including adolescent sexuality, substance abuse, teenage depression, violent behavior, activities preparation, attainment and maintenance of employment, and other social skills (Lovaas, 1987).

Social work will place more emphasis on prevention, a major issue to be considered, as the helping professions have a history of dealing with individuals only *after* they have exhibited problematic behaviors rather than *before* problematic behavior occurs. Some may wonder if we can really alter clients' behaviors after 20, 40, or 60 years of learning. Our task, therefore, is to facilitate the preventive and educative roles that can be assumed by social workers. We should develop criteria for early intervention. Prototypes of such an approach may be found in courses on parental effectiveness, sex education, marital enrichment, and so on. Such courses should focus on helping parents develop better communication and consistent child management skills, two variables research has shown are necessary conditions for successful child rearing (Hoffman, 1977), and helping prepare young adults for the requisites of marriage, with effective communication skills, problem-solving strategies, and conflict resolution procedures (Collins, 1971; Ely, Guerney, & Stover, 1973; Lederer & Jackson, 1968; Rappaport & Harrell, 1972; Satir, 1967). The use of behavioral techniques in preventive medicine is an exciting application of behavioral analysis. Prevention of coronary

181

heart disease is illustrated by efforts to identify high-risk individuals and apply behavioral techniques designed to decrease weight and increase exercise, stop smoking, and reduce serum cholesterol (Meyer & Henderson, 1974; Roskies, 1987).

We will have to evaluate how the different reinforcement strategies, i.e. cooperative or competitive, that schools employ affect the development of children's self-concepts and their attitudes toward adults in society, traditional societal values, norms, and institutions, and how they facilitate the development of relevant prosocial behaviors and a sense of belongingness in the child (Buckholdt & Wodarski, 1978; Hoffman, 1977).

MAINTENANCE AND GENERALIZATION OF BEHAVIORAL CHANGE

The incidence of family, child, and youth behavioral difficulties will continue to be a focus of preventive approaches. Evaluations of preventive practices based on traditional techniques are not encouraging. With the exception of programs based on the behavioral approach, little data exist to support practice efforts with families, children, and adolescents (Kazdin, Esveldt-Dawson, French, & Unis, 1987; Lovaas, 1987; Schinke, 1981; Wodarski & Bagarozzi, 1979). Even with the various behavioral programs, however, there remains yet the unresolved problem of the maintenance and generalization of behavioral change once achieved.

Maintenance can be viewed as the length of time between the termination of intervention and the continuance of the behavior. Generalization refers to the extent the behaviors learned in the clinical context occur at appropriate times, and to socially relevant people in the socially relevant settings. Thus, if the goal of a prevention program is for a child to develop adequate social and academic behaviors, then once these behaviors are acquired the crucial subsequent issues of maintenance and generalization must be addressed. The literature on maintenance and generalization indicates that these processes will not occur by chance, and, therefore, any sophisticated treatment program must directly address them (Epstein, Nudelman, & Wing, 1987; Kazdin, 1975, 1977; Koegel & Rincover, 1977; Stokes & Baer, 1977; Wahler & Graves, 1983).

Specific items involved in the maintenance and generalization of behavioral change are training relatives or significant others in the client's environment; training behaviors that have a high probability of being reinforced in natural environments; varying the conditions of training; gradually removing or fading the contingencies; using different schedules of reinforcement; using delayed reinforcement and self-control procedures, and so forth.

COGNITIVE FOCI

Cognitive theories propose, in their stages of development, that a child is in a concrete operations stage early in school and moves into more abstract, formal operational thought during adolescence. By utilizing cognitive-behavioral methods the worker is able to adjust the service mode according to the child's cognitive developmental stage. The ultimate goal of most cognitive intervention methods is to increase the individual's ability to control his/her own outcomes, with self-control being viewed as a developmental achievement that follows external control (Bugenthal et al., 1977). For adolescents, the achievement of adequate cognitive process is essential to their development of adequate self-concept and self-esteem.

Cognitive theorists have proposed several major approaches, many of which overlap. These approaches focus both on particular sets of cognitive deficits or ways in which thinking may deviate from the logical and on the methods by which these errors or deficits may be corrected. The ultimate aim in cognitive intervention is to produce change in the negative attitudes an adolescent has, thus reducing cognitive blocks to appropriate behavior.

Cognitive theorists' investigation of the client's thinking is based on two premises. First, clients think in an idiosyncratic way (that is, they have a systematic negative bias in the way they regard themselves, their world, and their future). Second, the way clients interpret events maintains their cognitive distortions.

Cognitive therapists view cognition in the treatment process as either the "behavior" that needs to be modified or as an area that is indirectly changed when the overt behavior is treated (Meichenbaum, 1975). The cognitive therapist attempts to alter what the adolescent thinks in order to effect a change in behavior. The belief is that therapy should aim at reducing the frequency of the cognitions that elicit the undesirable behaviors (Hulbert & Sipprelle, 1978). The focus is on the cognitive self-statements the client makes, and faulty self-statements are viewed as a result of a faulty belief system and thinking pattern (Meichenbaum, 1975).

Cognitive theorists believe there to be four types of cognitive distortions:

(1) Arbitrary inference: the process of drawing a conclusion when evidence is lacking or is actually contrary to the conclusion.

(2) Overgeneralization: the process of making an unjustified generalization on the basis of a single incident.

(3) Magnification: the propensity to exaggerate the meaning or significance of a particular event.

(4) Cognitive deficiency: the disregard of an important aspect of a life situation. Clients with this defect ignore, fail to integrate, or do not utilize information derived from experience, and consequently behave as though they have a defect in their system of expectations (Beck, 1970).

To address these distortions, the worker may have the client utilize problem-solving skills that are used throughout his/her life (Beck, 1976). In addition, a number of behavioral therapy procedures can be adapted to modify the cognitive self-statements (Meichenbaum, 1975). For example, cognitive theorists have emphasized the following cognitive aspects of depression. Beck (1976) assigned a primary position to a cognitive triad consisting of a very negative view of the self, of the outside world, and of the future. This triad is seen as the key to the consequences of depression, such as the lack of motivation, the affective state, and other ideational and behavioral manifestations. The depressed person's cognitions lead to misinterpretations of experiences; hence, many of the secondary responses are logical consequences of such misinterpretations. The depressed person is locked in an insoluble situation, the result of which is further despair (Calhoun, Adams, & Mitchell, 1974). Thus, cognitive responses that can be altered by the therapist are: (1) sense of hopelessness, (2) self-condemnation and self-defeating thoughts, (3) low self-esteem, (4) tension, (5) death wishes, and (6) sense of helplessness (Reynolds, 1985).

Significant interactive effects have been found to exist between the intervention approach and the person's attributional style (Bugenthal et al., 1977; Prager-Decker, 1980). The individual's expectations and assumptions will play a significant role in the success he/she will experience in therapy (Goldfried & Goldfried, 1975). In relation to success in therapy, Bandura et al. (1977) noted that regardless of the methods used, treatments implemented through the individual's actual performance achieve consistently superior results to those based on symbolic forms of the same approach.

SOCIAL NETWORKS

Data suggest that adolescents are at less social risk to develop mental distress if they are socially connected to other peers, i.e. social supports buffer stress, support and help individuals through crisis periods, promotes good physical health, and facilitates the acquisition and maintenance of relevant social competencies (Heller & Swindle, 1983; Thyer, 1987; Wahler & Graves, 1983).

One of the most perplexing yet critical problems confronting social work professionals interested in prevention is the effective use of networking for adolescents at risk. Questions that need to be resolved include the following. How can adolescents be tied to the networks available in their peer communities? What peer characteristics may be matched with adolescent attributes to facilitate networking and enhancement of the individuals' functioning? What support systems such as the church, extended family, and friends are available to enhance the adolescent's networks?

This aspect of prevention would involve development of programs to utilize efficacious and cost-effective assessment procedures to isolate physical, psychological, and social factors that lead to networking. Possible procedures include: (1) assessment of the adolescent's attributes such as homogeneity of peers, social cohesion, and services available; (2) enlistment of social networks and support groups such as family, peers, ministers, and significant adult models to provide necessary support; (3) preparation of the adolescent in terms of emphasizing appropriate social behaviors that will be rewarded and will facilitate integration into the social structure of their peer community; (4) educating the adolescent about support services available and whom to contact and gradually introducing the individual to appropriate available support systems; and (5) developing appropriate preventive intervention.

MACROLEVEL ANALYSIS

It is likely that future research will begin to unravel the complex relationship between societal experiences and prevention. How we can construct a society with macrolevel interventions as opposed to individual interventions to prevent or facilitate certain behavior has been virtually ignored by the field. For example, social policies with provision of incentives for welfare clients who can work to secure and maintain employment, designing physical environments in such a manner that the probability of criminal behavior is decreased, and so on must be examined. One example of an environmental design to facilitate the occurrence of a particular behavior is the "open schools" concept. In the open classroom the purpose is to increase social interaction among children and adults. The crucial questions center on how to structure environments that will support behavioral change achieved through interpersonal approaches, that is, provide enough reinforcers to maintain prosocial behavior, and what behaviors can be altered directly through macro-level intervention (Kelly, Snowden, & Munoz, 1977).

IMPLEMENTATION PREVENTION STRATEGY: WHERE, BY WHOM, WHY, HOW LONG, AND ON WHAT LEVEL?

Context of Behavioral Change

Unfortunately, if an adolescent exhibits a problematic behavior in one social context, such as school, the behavioral change strategies all too frequently are provided in another social context, such as a child guidance clinic, family service agency, or community mental health center. Such procedures create many structural barriers to effective intervention (Kazdin, 1977; Stokes & Baer, 1977). Data indicate that, if possible, preventive intervention should be provided in the same context where problematic behaviors are exhibited. If prevention change strategies are implemented in other contexts, the probabilities are reduced that learned behaviors can be sufficiently generalized and maintained.

Considerable study is needed to delineate those variables that facilitate the generalization and maintenance of behavior change. These may include choosing behaviors that will be maintained by the community support networks, substituting "naturally occurring" reinforcers, training relatives or significant others in the client's environment, gradually removing or fading contingencies, varying the conditions of training using different schedules of reinforcement, using delayed reinforcement and self-control procedures, and so forth (Kazdin, 1974, 1977). Such considerations equip workers in developing sophisticated and effective social service delivery systems which increase the probability of clients securing the necessary services to maintain themselves within their communities (Wodarski, 1980).

By Whom Should Change Be Delivered?

We have evidence to suggest that personal characteristics of social workers involved in prevention facilitate the delivery of services to clients. The worker should have similar attributes to facilitate the acceptance and subsequent participation in services provided (Ewing, 1974; Kadushin, 1972; Korchin, 1980; Thompson & Cimbolic, 1978). Other givens which research supports are: workers should be reinforcing individuals with whom adolescents can identify; they should possess empathy, unconditional positive regard, interpersonal warmth, verbal congruence, confidence, acceptance, trust, verbal ability, and physical attractiveness; and they should take time with adolescents and provide them the rationale for the services (Carkhuff, 1969, 1971; Carkhuff & Berenson, 1967; Fischer, 1975; Keefe, 1975; Lerner & Blackwell, 1975; Vitalo, 1975; Wells & Miller, 1973). Likewise, Bandura (1977), Rosenthal (1966), and Rosenthal and Rosnow (1969) have suggested that the worker's expectation of positive change in clients is also necessary. Additional research suggests that a behavioral change agent should have considerable verbal ability, should be motivated to help others change, should possess a wide variety of social skills, and should have adequate social adjustment (Berkowitz & Graziano, 1971; Gruver, 1971).

If the prevention worker chooses to employ an adolescent's parents, teachers, peers, or others as change agents, he/she must realize that they will have to assess at the very least how motivated these individuals are to help alleviate the dysfunctional behavior and how consistently they will apply preventive techniques, what means are available to monitor the implementation of prevention to insure that it is appropriately applied, and if the chosen change agent possesses characteristics such as similar social attributes, similar sex, and so forth that could facilitate the client's identification with him/her (Bandura, 1969, 1977; Banks, 1971; Berman, 1979; Berman & Rickel, 1979; Bryson & Cody, 1973; Tharp & Wetzel, 1969).

Rationale for Service Provided

The rationale for offering a prevention program should be based primarily on empirical grounds. The decision-making process should reflect that the workers have considered what type of agency should house the service, that they have made an assessment of the organizational characteristics of the treatment context, and that the interests of the agency personnel have been considered in planning the service. A number of additional questions should also be posited to insure the provision of relevant services. How can the program be implemented with minimal disruption? What new communication structures need to be used? What types of measurements can be used in evaluating the service? What accountability mechanisms need to be set up? What procedures can be utilized for monitoring the execution of the program (Feldman & Wodarski, 1974, 1976; Wodarski, 1981; Wodarski & Feldman, 1974)?

Duration

Few empirical guidelines exist regarding how long a service should be provided, that is, when client behavior has improved sufficiently in terms of quality and quantity, to indicate that services are no longer necessary. Such criteria should be established before the service is to be provided and these should indicate how the program will be evaluated. The criteria should enable workers to determine whether or not a service is meeting the needs of the client. Moreover, they should help reveal the particular factors involved in deciding whether or not a service should be terminated. The more complete the criteria, the less this process will be based on subjective factors. In answering such questions workers realize that theory, intervention, and evaluation are all part of one total interventive process in prevention.

Larger Units for Social Change to Effect Prevention

Even broadly defined social policy decisions can directly affect the behaviors that will be exhibited by clients. For example, certain economic policy decisions (e.g. those pertinent to teenage employment and education, housing, and other social phenomena) have a determinate effect on behaviors that clients will exhibit in the future. A decision to adopt a full employment policy will obviously affect clients. Likewise, a national children's rights policy would insure that each child is provided with adequate housing, education, justice, mental and social services, and so forth. Thus, the target for change may well be an institution or policy rather than the clients themselves.

If following a community analysis, a worker decides that a client *is* exhibiting appropriate behaviors for his/her social context and he/she determines that a treatment organization or institution *is not* providing adequate support for appropriate behaviors, or that it is punishing appropriate behavior, the prevention worker must then decide to engage in organizational or institutional change (Prunty, Singer, & Thomas, 1977). This may involve changing a social policy or a current bureaucratic means of dealing with people, or employing other strategies. In order to alter an organization, workers will have to study its components and assess whether or not they have the power to change these structures so that the client can be helped. In social work practice the primary focus has been on changing the individual. Future conceptualizations should provide various means of delineating how human behavior can be changed by interventions on multilevels (Wodarski, 1977). Thus, workers should learn that following such a framework of human behavior, an "inappropriate" behavior exhibited by a client must be examined according to who defined it as inappropriate and where requisite interventions should take place. The obvious question that will face the social worker is how to coordinate these multilevel interventions.

Interventions at the macro level are increasingly more critical in light of follow-up data collected five years later on antisocial children who participated in a year-long behavior modification program which produced extremely impressive behavioral changes in the children. Results indicate that virtually none of the positive changes were maintained (McCombs, Filipczak, Friedman, & Wodarski, 1978; McCombs, Filipczak, Rusilko, Koustenis, & Wodarski, 1977). Possibly, maintenance could be improved when change is also directed at macro levels which would provide the necessary support for changed behavior.

RESEARCH FOCI

Few would deny the controversy surrounding the efficacy of current social work preventive services aimed at changing adolescents' behavior. Issues pertain to where services should be provided and by whom, what is the proper duration of services, and where are appropriate criteria for evaluation. The legal emphasis on providing effective services to clients and the expressed desire to provide social services on an empirical and rational basis are motivating factors in the development of a sound theoretical base (Reid & Hanrahan, 1982; Wodarski, 1981; Wodarski & Bagarozzi, 1979a, 1979b).

Critical questions center on the following issues. What are the relevant human behavior variables that can provide a solid basis for structuring prevention services to adolescents? What guidelines can be furnished for structuring services from an organizational perspective? The development and implementation of adequate assessment procedures. What criteria can be utilized in the evaluation of services? How can one delineate the level of intervention of the micro-to-macro level continuum and the appropriate timing of the intervention to secure maximum benefits? Results and products culminating from a number of research projects over the last decade indicate rationale for a more elaborate comprehensive theory of prevention.

It is evident that more elaborate theories of human behavior are needed to provide the rationale for complex prevention systems that are based on principles derived from empirical knowledge, with the goal being to prevent adolescent dysfunctioning. These theories must consider biological, sociological, economic, political, and psychological factors as they interact in the human matrix to cause behavior (Wodarski, 1985). It is a definite challenge for any theory of human behavior to isolate those components that lead to prevention, such as the specific aspects of an intervention package in terms of expectations for change, role of cognitive processes, particular client and social worker characteristics, interventions, context of intervention, and so forth. Once this knowledge is developed, the choice of prevention techniques can be made on such criteria as client and worker characteristics, context of intervention, and type of intervention.

Recent evidence suggests that in order for prevention to be successful, macro-level intervention variables have to be considered. An adequate theory of prevention will isolate the social system variables (i.e. legal, political, health, financial, social services, educational, housing, employment, etc.) and their effects on human behavior. Moreover, these variables have to be addressed in a manner that focuses on the attainment of prevention and maintenance of behavior. Current theories fall far short of this goal.

Requisites for quality prevention research can be assessed in terms of cost and experimental design requisites in terms of the limitations and benefits of classical and time series designs for assessing prevention intervention.

SUMMARY

In the coming years we will witness more interventions with adolescents that take a preventive focus. This chapter has focused in on the following issues and how they relate to effective preventive services for adolescents: maintenance and generalization of behavioral change, cognitive foci, social networks, implementation prevention strategy, macro-level analysis, and research foci. The cost to adolescents from a social perspective and to our society from an economic perspective is substantial. If we do not utilize preventive interventions, we as a society will pay a great price.

REFERENCES

Bandura, A. (1969). *Principles of behavior modification.* New York: Holt, Rinehart & Winston.

Bandura, A. (1977). *Social learning theory.* Englewood Cliffs, NJ: Prentice-Hall.

Bandura, A., Adams, N., & Beyer, J. (1977). Cognitive processes mediating behavioral change. *Journal of Personality and Social Psychology, 35,* 125-139.

Banks, G. P. (1971). The effects of race on one-to-one helping interviews. *Social Service Review, 45*(2), 137-146.

Beck, A. (1970). Cognitive therapy: Nature and relation to behavior therapy. *Behavior Therapy, 1,* 184-200.

Beck, A. (1976). *Cognitive therapy and the emotional disorders.* New York: International Universities Press.

Berkowitz, B. P., & Graziano, A. N. (1972). Training parents as behavior therapists: A review. *Behavior Research and Therapy, 10,* 297-317.

Berman, J. (1979). Counseling skills used by black and white male and female counselors. *Journal of Counseling Psychology, 26*(1), 81-84.

Berman, S. F., & Rickel, A. U. (1979). Assertive training for low-income black parents. *Clinical Social Work Journal, 7*(2), 123-132.

Bryson, S., & Cody, J. (1973). Relationship of race and level of understanding between counselor and client. *Journal of Counseling Psychology, 20*(6), 495-498.

Buckholdt, D., & Wodarski, J. S. (1978). The effects of different reinforcement systems on cooperative behavior exhibited by children in classroom contexts. *Journal of Research and Development in Education, 12*(1), 50-68.

Bugenthal, D. B., Whalen, C. K., & Hienker, B. (1977). Causal attributions of hyperactive children and motivation assumptions of two behavior change approaches: Evidence for an interactionist position. *Child Development, 48,* 874-884.

Calhoun, K. S., Adams, H. E., & Mitchell, K. M. (1974). *Innovative treatment methods in psychopathology.* New York: Wiley.

Carkhuff, R. R. (1969). *Helping and human relations.* New York: Holt, Rinehart & Winston.

Carkhuff, R. R. (1971). Training as a preferred mode of treatment. *Journal of Counseling Psychology, 18,* 123-131.

Carkhuff, R. R., & Berenson, B. G. (1967). *Beyond counseling and therapy.* New York: Holt, Rinehart & Winston.

Collins, J. D. (1971). *The effects of the conjugal relationship modification method on marital communication and adjustment* (unpublished doctoral dissertation). The Pennsylvania State University.

Dangel, R. F., & Polster, R. A. (Eds.). (1984). *Parent training: Foundations of research and practice.* New York: Guilford.

Ely, A. L., Guerney, G. G., & Stover, L. (1973). Efficacy of the training phase of conjugal therapy. *Psychotherapy: Theory, Research and Practice, 10,* 201-207.

Epstein, L. H., Nudelman, S., & Wing, R. R. (1987). Long-term effects of family-based treatment for obesity on nontreated family members. *Behavior Therapy, 2,* 147-152.

Ewing, T. N. (1974). Racial similarity of client and counselor and client satisfaction with counseling. *Journal of Counseling Psychology, 21*(5), 446-449.

Feldman, R. A., & Wodarski, J. S. (1974). Bureaucratic constraints and methodological adaptations in community-based research. *American Journal of Community Psychology, 2,* 211-224.

Feldman, R. A., & Wodarski, J. S. (1976). Inter-agency referrals and the establishment of community-based treatment programs. *American Journal of Psychology, 4,* 269-274.

Fischer, J. (1975). Training for effective therapeutic practice. *Psychotherapy: Theory, Research and Practice, 12,* 118-123.

Goldfried, M., & Goldfried, A. (1975). Cognitive change methods. In F. Kanfer & A. Goldstein (Eds.), *Helping people change.* New York: Pergamon Press.

Gruver, G. G. (1971). College students as therapeutic agents. *Psychological Bulletin, 76,* 111-127.

Heller, K., & Swindle, R. W. (1983). Social networks, perceived social support, and coping with stress. In R. Felner, L. Jason, J. Moritsugu, & S. Farber (Eds.), *Preventive psychology: Theory, research and practice.* New York: Pergamon Press.

Hoffman, M. L. (1977). Personality and social development. In M. Rosenzweig & L. Porter (Eds.), *Annual review of psychology.* Palo Alto, CA: Annual Reviews.

Hulbert, R. T., & Sipprelle, C. N. (1978). Random sampling of cognitions in alleviating anxiety attacks. *Cognitive Therapy and Research, 2*(2), 165-169.

Jacobson, N. S., & Margolin, G. (1979). *Marital therapy: Strategies based on social learning and behavior exchange principles.* New York: Brunner/Mazel.

Kadushin, A. (1972). The racial factor in the interview. *Social Work, 17*(3), 88-98.

Kazdin, A. E. (1974). Effects of covert modeling and model reinforcement on assertive behavior. *Journal of Abnormal Psychology, 83,* 240-252.

Kazdin, A. E. (1975). *Behavior modification in applied settings.* Homewood, IL: Dorsey Press.

Kazdin, A. E. (1977). *The token economy.* New York: Plenum Press.

Kazdin, A. E., Esveldt-Dawson, K., French, N. H., & Unis, A. S. (1987). Problem-solving skills training and relationship therapy in the treatment of antisocial child behavior. *Journal of Consulting and Clinical Psychology, 55,* 76-85.

Keefe, T. (1975). Empathy and social work education: A study. *Journal of Education for Social Work, 11,* 69-75.

Kelly, J. G., Snowden, L. R., & Munoz, R. F. (1977). Social and community intervention. In M. Rosenzweig & L. Porter (Eds.), *Annual review of psychology.* Palo Alto, CA: Annual Reviews Inc.

Koegel, R. L., & Rincover, A. (1977). Research on the difference between generalization and maintenance in extra-therapy responding. *Journal of Applied Behavior Analysis, 10,* 1-12.

Korchin, S. J. (1980). Clinical psychology and minority problems. *American Psychologist, 35*(3), 262-269.

Lederer, W., & Jackson, D. (1968). *The mirages of marriage.* New York: Norton.

Lerner, R., & Blackwell, B. (1975). The GP as a psychiatric community resource. *Community Mental Health Journal, 11,* 3-9.

Lovaas, O. I. (1987). Behavioral treatment and normal educational and intellectual functioning in young autistic children. *Journal of Consulting and Clinical Psychology, 55*(1), 3-9.

McCombs, D., Filipczak, J., Friedman, R. M., & Wodarski, J. S. (1978). Long-term follow-up of behavior modification with high risk adolescents. *Criminal Justice and Behavior, 5,* 21-34.

McCombs, D., Filipczak, J., Rusilko, S., Koustenis, G., & Wodarski, J. S. (1977, December). *Follow-up on behavioral development with disruptive juveniles in public schools.* Paper presented at the 11th Annual Meeting of the Association for the Advancement of Behavior Therapy, Atlanta, Georgia.

Meichenbaum, D. (1975). Self-instructional methods. In F. Kanfer & A. Goldstein (Eds.), *Helping people change.* New York: Pergamon Press.

Meyer, A. J., & Henderson, J. B. (1974). Multiple risk factors reduction in the prevention of cardiovascular diseases. *Preventive Medicine, 3,* 225-236.

Prager-Decker, I. J. (1980). The efficacy of muscle relaxation in combatting stress. *Health Education, 11,* 40-42.

Prunty, H. E., Singer, T. L., & Thomas, L. A. (1977). Confronting racism in inner-city schools. *Social Work, 22*(3), 190-194.

Rappaport, A., & Harrell, J. (1972). A behavioral exchange model for marital counseling. *The Family Coordinator, 21,* 203-212.

Reid, W. J., & Hanrahan, P. (1982). Recent evaluation of social work: Grounds for optimism. *Social Work, 27*(4), 328-340.

Reynolds, W. M. (1985). Depression in childhood and adolescence: Diagnosis assessment, intervention strategies and research. In T. R. Kratochwill (Ed.), *Advance in school psychology* (Vol. 4) (pp. 133-189). Hillsdale, NJ: Lawrence Erlbaum.

Rosenthal, R. (1966). *Experimenter effects in behavioral research.* New York: Appleton-Century-Crofts.

Rosenthal, R., & Rosnow, R. L. (Eds.). (1969). *Artifact in behavioral research.* New York: Academic.

Roskies, E. (1987). *Stress management for the healthy type A: Theory and practice.* New York: Guilford Press.

Satir, V. (1967). *Conjoint family therapy.* Palo Alto, CA: Basic Books.

Schinke, S. P. (Ed.). (1981). *Behavioral methods in social welfare.* Hawthorne, NY: Aldine.

Schinke, S. P., & Gilchrist, L. D. (1984). *Life skills counseling with adolescents.* Baltimore: University Park Press.

Stokes, T. F., & Baer, D. M. (1977). An implicit technology of generalization. *Journal of Applied Behavior Analysis, 12,* 349-367.

Tharp, R. G., & Wetzel, R. J. (1969). *Behavior modification in the natural environment.* New York: Academic Press.

Thompson, R. A., & Cimbolic, P. (1978). Black students' counselor preference and attitudes toward counseling center use. *Journal of Counseling Psychology, 25*(6), 570-575.

Thyer, B. A. (1987). Community-based self-help groups for the treatment of agoraphobia. *Journal of Sociology and Social Welfare, 14*(3), 135-141.

Vitalo, R. L. (1975). Guidelines in the functioning of a helping service. *Community Mental Health Journal, 11,* 170-178.

Wahler, R. G., & Graves, M. G. (1983). Setting events in social networks: Ally or enemy in child behavior therapy? *Behavior Therapy, 14*(1), 19-36.

Wells, R. A., & Miller, D. (1973). Developing relationship skills in social work students. *Social Work Education Reporter, 21,* 60-73.

Wodarski, J. S. (1977). The application of behavior modification technology to the alleviation of selected social problems. *Journal of Sociology and Social Welfare, 4*(7), 1055-1073.

Wodarski, J. S. (1980). Procedures for the maintenance and generalization of achieved behavioral change. *Journal of Sociology and Social-Welfare, 7*(2), 298-311.

Wodarski, J. S. (1981). *Role of research in clinical practice.* Austin: PRO-ED.

Wodarski, J. S. (1985). *Introduction to human behavior.* Austin, PRO-ED.

Wodarski, J. S., & Bagarozzi, D. (1979a). *Behavioral social work.* New York: Human Sciences Press.

Wodarski, J. S., & Bagarozzi, D. (1979b). A review of the empirical status of traditional modes of interpersonal helping: Implications for social work practice. *Clinical Social Work Journal, 7*(4), 231-255.

Wodarski, J. S., & Feldman, R. A. (1974). Practical aspects of field research. *Clinical Social Work Journal, 2*(3), 182-193.

AUTHOR INDEX

SUBJECT INDEX